Working with Death and Loss in Shiatsu Practice

Working with Death and Loss in Shiatsu Practice

A Guide to Holistic Bodywork in Palliative Care

TAMSIN GRAINGER

Foreword by Richard Reoch

*Photographs by Anastazia Mac Corgarry
(www.littleredfoxes.co.uk)*

Illustrations by Janine van Moosel

Calligraphy by Alain Tauch

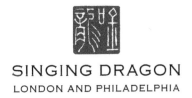

SINGING DRAGON

LONDON AND PHILADELPHIA

First published in 2020
by Singing Dragon
an imprint of Jessica Kingsley Publishers
73 Collier Street
London N1 9BE, UK

www.singingdragon.com

Library of Congress Cataloging in Publication Data
A CIP catalog record for this book is available from the Library of Congress

British Library Cataloguing in Publication Data
A CIP catalogue record for this book is available from the British Library

ISBN 978 1 78775 269 6
eISBN 978 1 78775 270 2

Printed and bound in Great Britain

To my ancestors

Contents

Foreword

Richard Reoch

When I first studied Shiatsu we were given an unnerving instruction to get down on the floor and start crawling over each other's bodies. Everyone suddenly got very nervous, incredibly embarrassed and awkward. It was one of our very first classes and none of us knew each other.

Our teacher took pity on us and said, 'If you can't do this with each other, just crawl on the floor like a little child, let your hands sink deeply into the carpet and let your whole being relax into our great mother, the Earth.'

The rich tapestry of this hands-on guide to working with death and loss in Shiatsu practice is often as direct, intimate and profound as that original instruction.

Describing the empathic work of a Shiatsu practitioner on a dying person, Tamsin tells the story of babies and small children who are acutely aware of the energy in the environment. As the practitioner holds the space, the vibrations of the treatment fill the room. The baby or the little child knows in their own being what is happening. Stopping what they are doing, they may crawl across the floor to be with the person who is lying there. In the presence of the deep Shiatsu work, the infant falls asleep. No longer required to be vigilant in the presence of death, she says, they can rest.

Whether it be this preverbal sensitivity of a small child or the silent energetic exchange of Shiatsu, both are deep listening. The one is led by the other. The other becomes inseparable from the one.

'I'll hold the rope while you scale the depths of the cavern,' said Edith Campbell, a chaplain to people diagnosed with HIV and AIDS in New York. Describing her work, she said, 'You are accompanying the person on a journey. You are travelling in unknown territory together.

What you are able to do is help clear the way so that person on the journey is able to tell you what they see, is able to point out to you the fullness and the beauty and the strangeness of the territory that they are going through.'

The rope, like the hands of the practitioner, is pliant. Moving and still at the same time, both are the conduits of human connectivity.

It is not that the practitioner or the chaplain are invincible. Quite the opposite. 'Let us be honest, death is a situation that many practitioners fear,' says Tamsin openly. 'However, Shiatsu practitioners also like to touch and be touched; we know it helps with life, and when our hands are in contact with a client, listening open-heartedly, we hear and recognize the suffering which is in all of us and cannot be ignored. As we give Shiatsu, the Ki moves back and forth between us, existing in the shared energetic field, and so it is inevitable that we exchange those feelings.'

It is in that field of energy – suffused with all our feelings, love and fear – that we learn profoundly from the dying and bereaved. Sometimes they 'hold the rope' for us.

When the great master Chu'ang Tzu was approaching death, his devoted students wanted to give him a large and expensive funeral. 'I shall have heaven and earth for my coffin,' he told them. 'All the planets and constellations will shine around me. What more could I need? Everything has been taken care of.'

It was as if he moved among them quietly, knelt down beside each one to place his hands upon their fearful and unsteady minds and offered them Shiatsu of the heart.

In that same way, this meticulous book is a work of love. May the treasures that it holds refresh, inspire and enrich the care we give to others and ourselves.

Richard Reoch
Author of Dying Well: A Holistic Guide
for the Dying and Their Carers

Acknowledgements

Over the years, I have identified my learning pattern: I watch and listen to my teachers, and read their work. Then I practise with myself and my clients (and talk about it to anyone who will listen). Often, I write about it, either notes in my journal, or an article or blog. I usually find that I pass it on through my classes and workshops in one form or another, and then I find that I can no longer identify it from the original. In fact, the older I get, the trickier it is to remember where I first came across something. In writing this book, I realized that I have blended and mixed, added and subtracted, and have likely bastardized as well. It has not been possible for me therefore to acknowledge every teacher at each juncture, and so I sincerely hope that those of you who recognize your ideas and teachings in these pages will know that I am honouring you rather than stealing or copying.

I therefore own it all and at the same time pay allegiance to those who inspired me and broadened my mind. It is a very long list because I have been at it quite a while and am a fervid reader. Here goes (in some sort of date order):

Sandra Reeves (and therefore Sonia Moriceau, who was her teacher, although I never met her) for my first Shiatsu sessions; Elaine Liechti, my first teacher, in whose Foundation classes I felt, 'I can do this', which was in direct contrast to the sense I had when I was learning to dance. Any teacher who can give their students that feeling is a great teacher; my colleague Cynthia Shuken – we met as students and have remained close. I am indebted to her and to Audicia Morley for her attention to detail, anatomical care, and creativity; Veet Allan for his book *Ocean of Streams* (1994); Bill Palmer; Nicola Pooley/Ley; Michael Rose; Anne Palmer, because in her inimitable way she was the gatekeeper to MrSS (membership of the professional register of the Shiatsu Society); Thea Bailey for being the only teacher I remember talking about death and for being a role model regarding cancer; I also gleaned common sense from Carol Dean about that subject; Suzanne Yates; Maria Serrano; Pauline Sasaki and Cliff Andrews; Jane Groombridge; Andrea Batterman for supervision and treatments; Laura Davison; Katharine Hall as a role model; Chris Jarmey; all the practitioners and teachers at the Women's Shiatsu Gatherings, particularly the meeting in Edinburgh, and Teresa Hadland for her friendship; Nick Pole (2017) for his book *Words That Touch*, his teaching and our lovely chats; Alice Whieldon for her luminous treatment/workshop at the European Shiatsu Congress in Vienna 2018; and Carola Beresford-Cooke for more than I can put into a single sentence, thank you.

Those who contributed to this book: Blanche Mulholland, Jane Groombridge, Richard Whiting, Jenny White, Liz Arundel, Diego Sanchez, Wilfried Rappenecker, Cliff Andrews, Bill Palmer, Elaine Liechti, Andrew Staib, Carol Shuford, Cat Westwood, Sarah Jane Churcher and Dan Keown.

For the artwork: Janine and her model, Anastazia, and especially Alain Tauch and Max Scratchmann.

For the editors, out of the kindness of their hearts: Andrew, Cynthia, Barbara, Irene, Isobel, Martin, Sally, Carola.

For the help and aid of all at Singing Dragon, especially Sarah, Maddy and Emma.

For the support of Dinah John, Jane Miller, Lesley Skeates, Ken Cockburn, Alice Cockburn, my mum, sister and brother and my dearest daughters, Alice and Isobel.

Going on a Journey into Death

Sit still. Settle. Close your eyes and let your electrons quieten. Draw in to Hara and wait. Exhale. Become aware of the pulsing of your blood, the timelessness of your fluids, the emptiness of your internal spaces. Shush. Listen. At a distance the world moves noisily. Your ears echo because of it. You are inside you. Only one. Small. Inhale.

Exhale. Underneath you, creatures nestle and wiggle, eat and excrete. Plant tendrils snake and root, cohabit. Water irrigates. Soil separates and refines.

Where are you from?   Inhale.

Exhale. Be between the Gate of Life (Ming men GV/Du 4) and the Sea of Qi (Qihai CV/Ren 6) where the umbilical cord of incarnation still throbs. You are a sentient being. Awake. Your eyeballs shift under your eyelids, your tongue is moistened by saliva, your metabolism jogs on. Feel life. Be enlivened.

To whom are you related?   Inhale.

Exhale. Leave through your crown. Rise up through the ceiling and the clouds, and in the realm of the sun, disperse. You are in the air. Let your trillions of cells float alone, allow them to list and tilt like a kestrel. On a draught of wind, be carried, easily. Watch what happens.

Where will you go when you die?   Inhale.

Exhale. Are you warm? Have the backs of your knees gone to sleep?

Can you move? With exquisite awareness, do you know the difference between each of your finger nails? Can you tell me your name? Inhale.

Exhale. Imagine you are lifting your hand and placing it on another person. Expand now – down, out, up. Sense the corners of the universe, the niches of your mind; open to the possibility of connection and communion; be willing.   Inhale.
    What do you feel?   Taste?   Smell?

Hear me ask you, how close is this person to life?   And when the answer comes, smile.   You exhale. Maybe they exhale, too.

Together you are in this moment. Sooner or later you will both re-enter the Universal River of Ki, each at your own time. Suddenly or slowly you will slip back into the stream of everything and nothing. You will recognize that place you came from, because it has been inside you all this time. It is the same in us all. Before – During – After. Formless, but full of potential you were. Released and having fulfilled it, you will be. Returning to the Source, you will have more experiences for an endless future.

Death is not about passing over, but going into. Right now, you are waiting to re-become. Meeting, once again, your basic essence you realize that we all were, are and will be unidentifiable from else, un-alone. Animal, vegetable, mineral, cosmic.

Know, in the Union of Ki, that this is true. As your awareness is speeding through electrical pathways, minute sensations arrest you. You stay. Focus a moment. When a sigh of recognition releases, on you travel. Silently, without time, and yet here at the same time as otherwhere. You both understand any meaning which is necessary. Wordless, the two of you discover that life and death are really the same Ki. If one of you is ready, the other may accompany them some of the way to say goodbye, until the next meeting.

Exhale. Your hand lifts away from the other person. Now the exchange has taken place it cannot be undone. Her imprint is on you and yours on her. You will not forget. You carry that. You walk away, stepping on. You stop, turn, smile.

Breathing onwards. How can you translate to the grieving that was inhabited, that was so real and clear? How to console and reassure? Perhaps you remain with the living and the dead simultaneously ∞ a link. You know it is possible to be whole O even now. Inhabit this and you will offer succour to others.

* * *

Shiatsu cares for the whole: the physical, emotional, mental and spiritual. It is especially suited to work with death and loss. Our skills are so broad that we can touch and teach, listen and speak; we provide a bridge spanning both banks (what are known as life and death) and, more importantly, the space between. What we have now, this amalgamation of Eastern and Western medicine, philosophy and sensibility, is indeed unique. The intelligence with which we sit with another, our ability to transcend earth and remain grounded, fly with spirit, and at the same time know our centre, is immensely special and valuable.

Let us look again at our place in all things, that we may inspire and expire in peace.

Introduction

Of course, I cried while I wrote this book. It was an appropriate response. Even though I thought that an event had already been grieved for and dealt with, I still cried when I remembered it again. It is said that grief never ends, it just changes, and that bit by bit we get used to it, and it is true that there have always been new aspects to the losses I have suffered, different versions conjured by my memory, and alternative perspectives depending on my age and recent experiences. I remember when a friend died leaving two young daughters, I feared that I, too, might die and leave my children motherless. Now that they are older, I am relieved and thankful to be alive to watch them grow up, and my awareness is focused on letting them go their own way, something my friend did not have the chance to try. I knew that Shiatsu was supporting me in a way that no other therapy or medication could.

Eight years earlier, my family and I had collected at my father's bedside in the Heart of Kent hospice. Wordless, he lay still as we remembered and prepared ourselves for life without him. We did not know if he could hear us or whether he knew we were there. Alone with him through the following night, I recalled his confidence in his religious faith, and, as the hours passed, I sensed his spirit in that liminal place, flitting from here to there, and back, acclimatizing, slowly releasing. We said adieu. I had not acknowledged until then that Traditional Chinese Medicine (TCM) and Zen theory had offered me a precious template both for my personal use and to share with others in my work.

In 2015, I became more and more aware that my previous zest and enthusiasm for life had waned. I kept hearing these internal questions: 'If I die tomorrow, will I be where I want to be, will I have done what I want to do?' With the aid of my family, friends, Shiatsu colleagues and other therapists, I slowly released myself from some responsibilities and took a sabbatical. It was while I was walking the Camino in Spain that I decided to write an article on the way I taught about death and loss at The Shiatsu School Edinburgh (established 2000) where I was Director and Principal Teacher. For years, I had fitted it into the curriculum which I was accredited to follow by the Shiatsu Society (UK). And that was the seed from which this book grew.

Over and over again, in the process of writing, I read this phrase: 'We avoid talking about death.' In fact, my research belies that. There are not only thousands of books, blogs and articles available, but sell-out Death Cafes (yes, you can discuss death while taking afternoon tea!), theatre, conference and pop-up events, plus social media accounts with thousands of followers (Death Salon: 28,000 followers on Instagram; Natural Death Centre: 17,000 followers on Twitter). I have come across countless, wonderful examples of writing about grief and loss in libraries, bookshops and online. I have heard some inspirational dialogue about end-of-life care in conferences, debates and on the radio – people speaking eloquently about life and living, fears, sharing their suffering, and detailing the sort of death they wish for themselves and those they love. I found that one link led to the next; one woman's thoughts had clearly inspired another's; and I discovered a whole body of literature and personal experiences spread out before me.

In the clinic, however, it has been a different matter. There, healthy clients do not often broach the subject. If death or loss come into my mind in a session, then as a practitioner I find a way to open up a conversation and it is usually the beginning of an interesting exchange. But, do they initiate? Very rarely. I am not sure why – they could be uneasy about mentioning it in the Shiatsu context, maybe they cannot, or simply do not want to. I do find that those who are close to dying make passing reference to the fact with comments like 'In the time I have left…' and '…because I do not have much time'. It is always hanging in the air.

What this has shown me is that Shiatsu is coming to maturity at exactly the time when health services around the world are starting to need what we offer as part of their palliative care policy. Increasingly, their reports contain language which is familiar to us – that death is a natural part of life and that care for the dying must be holistic. The World Health Organization (2019a) states: 'Palliative care…affirms life and regards dying as a normal process; intends neither to hasten or postpone death; integrates the psychological and spiritual aspects of patient care.' Where have we heard that before? Between us, we have the expertise to demonstrate and communicate how our multi-levelled approach is exactly what patients are asking for – to find the balance between living well right up to the point of death, and preparing themselves and their loved ones for what comes after. For death focuses the mind.

There was one Shiatsu practitioner in the UK who started this dialogue many years ago in what was, then, an unusual setting, Thea Bailey (1999). As one of the team who was instrumental in starting up the Bristol Cancer Care Centre (now Penny Brohn Cancer Care[1]) in England, with doctors and other medical staff as well as complementary therapy colleagues, Bailey also ran workshops for her fellow therapists which many attended, as I did. In 1997, the complementary health publisher Gaia Books published *Dying Well – A Holistic Guide for the Dying and Their Carers* (1997) by British trained practitioner, Richard Reoch, to quiet acclaim. His book is based on Buddhist principles and contains some beautiful ideas and advice. Reoch writes: 'It takes love, patience and the support of an open heart to do "everything possible" for a person on the threshold of death's transformation' (p.52). *Working with Death and Loss in Shiatsu Practice* does not espouse any particular religious or spiritual direction, although it acknowledges that many Shiatsu practitioners have a shared Taoist background and entirely agrees with these open-hearted attitudes.

The best known, non-Shiatsu texts on the subject of grief and dying come from the valuable work of Dr Elisabeth Kübler-Ross, psychiatrist, humanitarian and hospice pioneer. She is well respected in medical and complementary circles alike, and wrote, 'To work with the dying patient requires a certain maturity which only comes from experience. We have to take a good hard look at our own attitude toward death and dying before we can sit quietly and without anxiety next to a terminally ill patient' (2019, p.269). This book is an invitation to become aware of this, to open up compassionately to our feelings. It suggests that we enquire within and sit with our fears in the belief that our clinical work will benefit from the process.

Today, in the UK, US, Australia and New Zealand, there is a dedicated group of Shiatsu practitioners working in hospitals, hospices

---

1   Penny Brohn UK, Living Well with Cancer UK: https://www.pennybrohn.org.uk

or hidden away in private practice, and work is currently under way to document and unite us. Often unpaid, the work is perhaps by its nature humble. In addition, most practitioners bring their skills to the aid of families and friends in the face of death and illness. Many of these colleagues have kindly contributed their experiences and advice.

This book explores the myriad ways in which we as practitioners and our clients meet death. It examines good practice and suggests how to engage with clients to enable them to be sustained through that experience. It looks at the intersection with illness, but does not go into detail about physical symptoms, diseases and how to treat each individual one. Rather, it will focus on the practitioner's preparation for this type of work, and the emotional, mental and spiritual aspects of working with clients who are dealing with grief, bereavement and loss, facing a terminal illness, or dying. It is about the sorts of reactions people have if they are grieving, shocked, scared or angry in the face of death and its threat.

One way or another, we are all managing the dying process every day, as well as dealing with the death which is constantly around us – among the people we know and in the media. The list of how and when we come across this topic in our work is long, so the chances are that you will either be dealing with it right now, in your practice, or will have done so at some time in the past. In the nine chapters of this volume there are a wide range of situations: from young people who may be facing death 'before time'; to people considering suicide; those who are dicing with death through alcohol or drug dependency; and people living with chronic illness who are familiar with the loss of physical ability, control and maybe of contact with colleagues. There are sections on grief throughout, as it relates to the familiar theories (TCM, the Five Elements and Zen Shiatsu) and its features and associated behaviours.

Those of us who practise Shiatsu believe it can help those who are suffering or scared, in shock or in a traumatic state. The parasympathetic nervous system triggers the relaxation response, and Shiatsu seems to have an effect on this, which might explain our popularity in a medical environment at the end of life. We aim to facilitate appropriate emotional release without the need to ask searching questions; reduce fear and anxiety levels; and dissipate anger and frustration which are very often around after someone has died. Our clients tell us that Shiatsu raises their awareness and aids self-management and empowerment in taking responsibility for their wellbeing. My personal enquiry shows that Shiatsu is well placed to support and benefit clients who are facing death.

Any book that purports to be an aid for working with people who are facing death must attempt to arm the reader with useful information to enable them to enter the institutions where these people are, reassure their friends and relatives, and support an understanding of death, grief and loss in the community. You may be searching for a surety, for a definitive answer to: 'What do I do if my client is dying?' There is none! Although there are lots of ideas and suggestions. You do know what to do, you have the skills, but, if you are not in contact with that inner knowledge – and fear does have a tendency to disconnect us from such feelings – the questions contained here will trigger your thoughts and stimulate you to enquire into your core beliefs so that you can find your innate talents in this area.

Working with Death and Loss in Shiatsu Practice is not research-based; that is, what is written here is not the result of trials and studies using large cohorts and with extrapolated data. Instead, it is the accumulated knowledge from my 30 years as a Shiatsu practitioner in private practice and corporate settings, and as a teacher at The Shiatsu School Edinburgh, with health visitors, at the Scottish Office and in tertiary education. It addresses the underlying theory with specific regard to the spirit at death and the movement of Ki in associated states. It has energy exercises, a section on preparation for the practitioner's own death (insurance, the law and keeping of records), multiple ways of working with clients, and a guide to supervision, mentoring, co-counselling and other aids to self-development.

There is a section for teachers who may be working with a student who is dying or dies and who then continues to work with the deceased's peers. If you are called on to write an obituary or contact that deceased student's family, you can refer to that part. Finally, there are plans for classes that focus on death and dying as a valuable and necessary part of an under- or postgraduate training programme. Please note also that any case studies used have been anonymized to protect identity.

Although I am a Zen Shiatsu practitioner, I also have considerable experience with Movement Shiatsu, Barefoot Shiatsu, the Extraordinary Vessels and Seiki on which I draw. I have endeavoured to give examples from as many styles of Shiatsu as I can, so that the book is useful to you whatever you practise. These are ideas and are not intended to be the definitive way to do something – there are more possibilities 'in heaven and earth' than can be thought of in the writing of one book! I encourage you to find your own way of working with clients and students in this field, either drawing on your own teaching and experience or making it up yourself, but I hope you will find stimulation here.

While I have attempted to acknowledge my limitations and asked others to fill those gaps – for which I am very grateful and you have been named – there are also some places I did not go. I have not referred to giving Shiatsu to animals even though some practitioners must work with those who are dying. I do not have enough experience to start writing about that. Neither do I write extensively about off-body or light body work, although I have mentioned it in contexts where I have used it to effect or where it seems particularly apposite. Some styles of Shiatsu are mentioned but I do not elaborate, as there are fine books on those subjects, and, in general, I have assumed that my readers will have a working knowledge of the other modalities based on my teaching, assessing (on behalf of the Shiatsu Society, UK) and research of the initial Shiatsu training in Europe, the US and Australia.

I have aimed to use language which is as inclusive as possible. I have tended to avoid the verb 'to treat' or the word 'treatment'. These do come to mind because many of us use them, but they also have connotations of the medical – 'I am treating her with diazepam' – and of a hierarchical relationship between practitioner and client which many of us continue to question. In Shiatsu, we sometimes employ the term 'self-healing' ('I am doing Amuku for self-healing'), but not the word 'healing' on its own to describe a result ('my client said she felt healed'). I do not make the claim that Shiatsu heals people, and I do not train practitioners to be healers.

I have researched diverse attitudes to death and dying around the world to recognize the many cultures which make up our client groups. I looked into the history of death ritual and belief in differing religions and practices, and realized that to cover them all deeply and with adequate respect necessitates a separate book (Murray Parkes *et al.* 2015).

The true depth and efficacy of Shiatsu lies in a pure and mindful touch. The skilled practitioner has the ability to sink into a place where knowledge and experience are trusted and fully integrated, such that the courage to *be*, to co-exist with the client, can be accessed. We all deal with variations on the theme of death in our work, and it can take courage and strength to look at them. When we practise that rigorous observation, we are developing the ability to touch in just the right places without denying any of the client's experience. At one and the same time we are also being open to our own recognition of death in life.

Tamsin Grainger

Please share your experience working with those who are dying and your practice. Contribute to the discussion here: http://shiatsu.ryoho. co.uk/new-book-working-with-death-and-loss-in-shiatsu-practice.

Disclaimer: There is reference to law (from the EU, UK, US, Australia, New Zealand and Canada) in the book. All details are correct at the time of publication.

— Chapter 1 —

Overview of Death and Loss

This chapter starts with death! It defines death and why it exists. It looks at why we fear it so much, the language used to describe it, and how those words and phrases reflect our underlying feelings. It is about shared language and an understanding about death in the therapeutic context. There is some underlying theory and we will examine how that affects the practitioner. In subsequent sections, you will find these topics elucidated in more detail and different contexts.

Saying death out loud

I am a white, middle-class British woman brought up in the Christian tradition of the Church of England. My background, upbringing, teaching and personality have resulted in my tendency to name things so that they are not hidden. I have a reputation for directness and I suspect that what underlies that is the hope that these things can be faced, and perhaps released or better understood, as long as they do not cause distress to others. I have fears and worries about death, as many people do, but I would still prefer to say the word *death* out loud, so that it is in the common space to be shared and acknowledged. The title I always used when planning the training timetables for my school in Edinburgh was *Shiatsu and Death*.

As time went on, however, and without realizing it, I noticed I was starting to use a different word. I understood, in a subtle and gradual way, that the word death was unacceptable. I would say it to someone in a discussion, but when they repeated it back to me, they substituted the phrase *passed away*; or when I overheard a student being asked what they did at a recent class, they would say, 'You know, about loss and stuff'. The word *grief*, I learned, is okay to use, and *end of life* is a phrase which is now widely employed, particularly in the hospice movement. In fact, that term, *end of life*, is very much the buzz phrase as I write, but not *death*.

Yes, things are changing. There is a great deal of time and money being spent, a great many books being published, and information about death and dying springing up all over the place. The Death Project,[1] The Art of Dying Well,[2] Dying Matters[3] – death is on the television, radio, all over the internet, and increasingly on people's lips. Across the English-speaking world, organizations and conferences are being held, bringing together specialists in 'ante-mortem, peri-mortem and post-mortem' (to use terms from the Death Salon).[4] Although Shiatsu practitioners have been working with clients with life-threatening illness and managing chronic disease, have been sitting with the dying and supporting the grieving for a very long time, it is in this 21st-century context of revealing the once hidden that this book has found its place.

In the UK and US, you have been able to hear cancer being colloquially referred to as *the C word* for quite a while. Now we hear people speak of *the D word* as well. Using that phrase is a way of adding seriousness to death, and at the same time avoiding using the actual term. For it is not just that society in general seems to love abbreviations, but that in this case there is a Difficulty with saying the word Death! It seems too Direct, too rough, too much like straight-talking. It is sometimes argued that it is upsetting to be asked, 'Has your dad *died* now?' 'When did your aunt *die*?' Or 'Did your client *die* of cancer?' It turns out that for some people, it is also upsetting to be the poser of those questions. We are shy about naming something so final, something that may have been a most painful thing. Some of us even worry that in naming death we attract it.

Fear of death

So, we do not call death by its own name. Why not? Above, I suggested that it may have something to do with the pain we think we may have to endure, what has been described by Chan and Chow (2006, synopsis) as 'the fear which marks the boundary between the known and unknown'.

---

1 https://susanbriscoe.wordpress.com
2 www.artofdyingwell.org
3 https://www.dyingmatters.org
4 https://deathsalon.org

It is not uncommon for Chinese people to believe that haunting by evil spirits would be the result of talking about death. We human beings are very complex and there are many influences on the way we think and act. We suffer from a great deal of trepidation and even horror about this unknown future. Philip Larkin (2012, pp.115–116), a British poet, writes of the dread, the terrible and true certainty of nothing after we die. It overcomes and stalls him in the early hours of the morning. Yeats (n.d.), the Irish poet, questioned what will happen to him, conjuring in his writing a naked, stricken and punished existence after death.

What is death?

Lucretius (2015) called it 'the icy pause of life'. Medically and scientifically, death is the permanent cessation of breath and physical functioning of the vital organs. On the emotional, mental and spiritual levels, we stop feeling, thinking and relating to the Godhead or to anything 'bigger' than us because these things are reliant on the brain, heart and spirit being physically alive.

In Chapter 2, we will take an in-depth look at the Traditional Chinese Medicine, Five Element and Zen Shiatsu approach. However, the theory is less important to us as human beings than the practicality – the before and after of death. Other than making the choice about what should happen to our body, most of us find the process of dying, what happens to the spirit or soul and the impact our death might have on others afterwards, more pressing. If we are not the one dying, the crucial thing is initially how we will manage to be with the person who is, and how we will cope without them. For Shiatsu practitioners, it is even more complicated, because we are in a power relationship with our clients, and that brings with it questions of responsibility. Such things are the concern of this book.

Cycle of life

In Ancient Greece, it was believed that when the Fates decided time was up, your corpse took on the shape of the former person and separated from the soul. They believed that the soul was the end reason for being, the essence of you, and that therefore death was a form of change, not a final ending. There was, however, disagreement about the detail: Aristotle said the soul was 'the form of the living thing', that everyone had one and it was inseparable from us, whereas Plato believed it was divisible.

Shiatsu practitioners are conversant with Yin and Yang: we are trained to compare one thing to another and not deal with absolutes, seeing life from a cyclical point of view, and knowing that in one thing there is always its counterpart. However, when it comes to death, we can still find ourselves thinking in that linear and 'logical' way. Fear can do that: it can change a usually open mind into a tunnel (and not the sort of tunnel through which many of those who have had near death experiences report that we go at the end – the one that ends in a white light!). We know some of the possible explanations of what happens after we die: there is at least one per religious group, plus other versions too, based on science, dreaming, meditation, stories and intuition. Despite there being so many accounts of similar experiences that it is tempting to give them credence, we are still scared, and in this we are like our clients. If we take a good look at our collective avoidance of death, we might deduce that it is a big, bad thing. We hold on, we do not let go without a fight, for all the world as if death were the enemy. We forget that there is no life without death. We know it, but we spend a lot of time, energy and money trying to stop it, or at least put it off.

Let us go back a moment.

One of the wonders of our Shiatsu training is the first year when we are introduced to the Five Elements. One by one, we are immersed in the separate parts of the natural cycle, identifying with each, until we come back to the start and view all five as a whole. It is then that we begin to look at the relationships between them and it all makes such sense. As time goes by, we learn to appreciate each season, *all* the colours, *all* the tastes and smells and sounds, and although we will always have more to learn, it is hoped that we do not get to the end without deeply understanding the symbiosis, and having absolute certainty in their mutual coexistence.

Then we move out into the world of practice and we teach our clients and students, as we ourselves were taught, how necessary it is to breathe out, as well as in. We remind ourselves, each time that we sit beside a client before the first touch, to release our muscles and internal fascia, because we know that our tendency is to hold on ('I let my shoulders relax, I let my hips sink down'). We are all about balancing the Ki and supporting it to flow. More, we know that stagnation occurs if we cease moving; that resisting change would be going against nature herself; and that without winter there will be no spring.

There are not so many complementary therapists who work in this way; it is one of the unique things about us – our work with the natural cycles of nature and of the human body means that we know the necessity for death. We might struggle against it personally, and think it is a failure if we succumb to it, we might feel the same surge of love for life if we are personally faced with it, but we do know, deep down, that it must happen. For the cycle of life to keep turning, there must be death.

If we approach our clients with this knowledge, if we have integrated it such that we honestly practise it, our presence will be invaluable when we visit a dying client or lay a warm hand on a grieving relative. If we know and accept this in our cells, it will affect our tone of voice, clients will see it in our eyes, and feel it in the Ki field all around the futon, table or stool. At one and the same time, that acceptance of the inevitable and rightness of death will serve to reassure. It will acknowledge the suffering, for it is impossible for any of us to meet death without meeting, too, the terrible, aching loss. Once known, it is not forgotten, and if we allow that experience to exist, find a way to *live with death*, we will be able to do great service to others.

Of course, it is not true that all Shiatsu practitioners think the same thing, despite the theory that underpins what we do. We have knowledge born from working with Ki and we know that a great deal of what we were taught and have read is true a lot of the time – we hear and see it in sessions. One client points to a spot and tells us what it feels like, surprising us by using exactly the same words we learned to associate with that Tsubo when we were studying. Another traces a 'line' where she feels a sensation and it is precisely a meridian we can show her on the chart. It might follow, then, that some of us believe the ancient texts and are convinced that we merely *shift across* at death and continue in another form. If we do, it makes our job a little easier. The Ki born of such certainty results in a simplicity and effectiveness of being with, and touching, a dying client or someone who is facing death.

Other practitioners, however, believe that each individual is unique, and therefore the possibilities about what happens at death are too. For them it is the Zen aspect of being in the moment that is the truth. Each encounter is a new one and each client must be met with *Beginner's Mind*. Then there are practitioners who are altogether unsure, and there are those who follow a clear, religious belief or set of precepts – when it comes to this we are as varied as the rest of the human population.

Language and terminology

Now we must ask, will the TCM or religion, or both, allied with clinical practice, be enough to sustain us as we accompany family members or clients through *the final gateway*?

In that question, I used a metaphor for death – the final gateway – and that brings us back to language and how we speak about grief, loss and death. Our clients very often refer to certain body parts using metaphors rather than anatomical words, and if they are generally understood or shared in the community, that may do very well. The same is true about death: there is a series of familiar similes or phrases that we use with those close to us, including our friends, phrases such as 'passed away', 'moved across', 'gone to a better place' and 'she is now an angel in heaven'. It may be that we choose our friends exactly because we recognize that we have a shared language when we first meet them. However, if the same happens in a Shiatsu session, if you or your client use a euphemism or a word which is open to interpretation, then it can cause problems, and it is vital that our reciprocal communication facilitates mutual comprehension and not confusion.

Many of us will hear stories of children who are told, 'Mummy has stepped out', or, 'Your dad has passed away', by another parent, a well-meaning relative, a teacher or other adult. We may have even been told a similar thing ourselves when we were younger, or have spoken like this to our own children. It is not surprising that some young people become confused as a result, because there are alternative meanings to these phrases. Mummy has stepped out where? Of the room? Into the garden? How has dad passed away? What does that mean? In these types of circumstances, the children can be forgiven for not knowing where their parent has gone or if that person will come back again. The confusion arises because the adults know what they mean by those phrases and the children do not.

In Shiatsu practice, it can be useful to stay with the language that the client uses, but there are pitfalls with this too. There is a comfort in shared understanding, and it may be very important that the client feels comfortable when all around them is painful or upsetting. To use recognized phrases puts someone at their ease and helps them relax, aiding bonding. It also shows respect, acknowledging that these are the words they have chosen, in the same way that we would use the touch which they prefer.

The ways a client chooses to describe what has happened to him, or what he is scared might happen, are in any case valuable. The words they choose convey a world of information about them and their background and we can learn much from hearing how he speaks about death. He not only reveals something of his inner self, but gives us an idea which elements, organs or meridians are at play and what we might do to support him.

Alternatively, he could be using language he thinks we want to hear or that he hopes we will find acceptable. He could be using what he has been taught when really he wants to say something different. This might be because someone else has given him the message that he should or should not say certain things in certain situations. Matters of life and death might therefore be times when the spoken word, talking about or asking how the topic was spoken about when he was growing up, could be appropriate.

BB was in the final days of his life and in our initial conversation he expressed the belief that he would disappear, and he waved his arms outwards from his upper body. 'You will disappear,' I repeated back to him, copying his tone of voice, which went down at the end of the word disapp*ear*, and his gesture, as accurately as I could. 'Yes,' he replied, 'I have had my time and in a little while I will go.' With this he changed to his left arm only and made a movement with it as if he was wiping things off a table. *Disappear* and *go* had different connotations to me and I wanted to be sure I understood – did he believe that he would become as air, for example, that he would move on to somewhere else, or even that he would be moved away, as if someone else was clearing him up? So I used both his phrases, one after the other: you will disappear, you have had your time and in a little while you will go (with accompanying and mirrored body gestures). His eyes turned inwards and he stopped breathing as loudly. I waited. What followed was a filming over of tears, a shuddery breath, and when he looked up at me he whispered, 'I won't be here any more', and he opened out both palms beside him.

Sitting still and quietly acknowledging his Ki, feeling the reverberations in my own system, my heart opened as his hands had done and I let the wave of sorrow move through me. In these immediate moments, the Shiatsu was just this – his Ki and my Ki meeting, mingling in the air. I recognized that my Ki was moving up the centre line of my chest and into my throat and head, and that there was a dispersing quality to it. I saw the details of his body, saw it change in response to his inner feelings – the dichotomy between a gratefulness in the loosening of his previously tense shoulders and also the sinking, letting go of his chest and Hara, the blanching of his face from the inevitability of it all. This was Shiatsu without the body-to-body touch. Our awareness, my mindfulness and his honesty meant that his Ki was being met and could change.

This example highlights the exquisite variation of words to describe not just what might happen to us when we die, but also how we feel about it and the implications.

We can say, 'I like to use the words death, grief and loss because they are unequivocal, how does that sound to you?' Or we can simply go ahead and use the words we personally like to use, even if they are different from the client's, as a test, to see if our hunch is correct, and see what reaction they have. If we are working with clients through an interpreter because we do not speak their language, or if they are speaking English but it is not their native tongue, it will be even more important to comprehend carefully.

Touch, a universal language

We are lucky that the language of touch, and of Ki, is universal. If there is not a shared, spoken vocabulary, then we can use this other way to communicate, together with our sense of utmost respect for the human condition. After all, suffering is suffering wherever it is found around the world.

Let us look at why clients seek us out. Some may have focused initially on a physical problem. In the same way that most patients go to their general practitioner for physical issues in the first place, this is perhaps easier and more familiar. Then, in its unravelling, it might turn out that the physical symptoms are related to grief and loss. As practitioners, we might have guessed or known that early on, perhaps because of our theory (the connection between the Metal element and grief), because of their breathing patterns (the Lung and melancholy), or because of our understanding of embodied pathology (lung disease and sadness), but the client might not have been aware of it. Then the question we ask ourselves is whether we name it, or whether we just touch and see what happens. Do we say that those symptoms can be related to grief (thereby opening the subject in words), or do we touch and see if they make their own connection? These are decisions each of us has to make for ourselves and they guide our practice and the way we relate to our clients. What is important here is that we may want or need to say the word *death* out loud.

What we believe about death

Our beliefs about what happens to us after we die and the rituals surrounding death are varied and complex. If we identify as Christian, Muslim or another type of religion, the way we talk about these things will follow the scriptures or teachings of that way, and working with clients within the same community will be simple because we will share a certain approach. We may choose to declare this on our publicity, thereby attracting others of the same faith. Around the world, we find multiple faiths with diverse approaches: this book will not go into any one of them in detail. Suffice to say that Shiatsu practitioners must either be inclusive and open-minded, or state clearly what their specific beliefs are in order to avoid insult or unlawful behaviour. Having a religious or spiritual context for death can be reassuring and stabilizing. Statistics show that those who believe in some sort of God are less likely to be fearful or to be searching for the reason why, and are more accepting of their fate (Jong *et al.* 2017). However, there are some who lose their previously stalwart faith when faced with the end of life, and this can leave a client in more distress than would be experienced by an atheist, who is clear that they do not believe in anything, or an agnostic, who knows that they do not know if there is or is not a God to believe in.

Conclusion

As Shiatsu practitioners, we aim to use a simple touch. We know how important the work of the mind is and we try to align our intention with our actions. Whether we are using a prescribed technique or working more from intuition, we like to empty our mind, focus on the Ki of the two of us, and make contact, with clarity. It follows, then, that we tend to favour clear and straightforward communication as well, and when working in this field, we must choose the language that is both comfortable for us and does the job allotted to it. In the course of taking a case history for a new client, and indeed if we have been working with someone for a long time, we may well be told of someone's death, and so it is necessary to have a way to speak about this topic with the same accuracy with which we touch.

The word *death* is unequivocal, but in Western society it may cause alarm or shock, and it is useful that we discuss and reflect on that in order to avoid any misunderstandings. Language is important, and our clients' choices reflect their underlying feelings. First, we examine our beliefs and experiences about death, then decide what words and beliefs suit us as individual practitioners. Once that has happened, we will be using these terms and ideas with awareness, and our clients will benefit from that.

— Chapter 2 —

Theory and Practical Shiatsu

This chapter looks at Shiatsu theory as it pertains to death and loss. It looks at the older ideas as well as at current practice, all from the perspective of the end of life and its consequences. It does not constitute a full introduction or explanation of Shiatsu and its theoretical origins. Each section uses language and terminology which must be familiar to the reader in order to be understood, and, to that end, there is a glossary at the back of the book if you need to remind yourself of the terminology.

In situations where the client cannot lie down on the futon or a massage table, the session may take place in a chair or wheelchair, or the client may have wires and tubes connected to her, reducing the body surface area available to touch. Reaching the back surface can be especially tricky. Perhaps the sides have to be up on the hospital bed, maybe the wheelchair has all sorts of gadgets attached to it, or it could be that you would like to minimize any potentially invasive movement for the sake of calm. In all of these situations, practitioners must be resourceful and flexible in their methods of diagnosis, techniques and ways of tuning into the Ki.

Ki

I prepare myself carefully when I work with clients who are facing death. I do not know what will happen, what their Ki will feel like or how much will be asked of me, but I do know that I want mine to be centred and grounded. As the practitioner, I wait for my Ki to settle, taking plenty of time to be present (see Figure 2.1). Stillness, a relaxed alignment, self-awareness and acknowledgement of what is happening are important. I have decided to be with this person for the duration. I want him to know that he has the choice. We wait. We are setting up our own energetic space, coming into resonance with ourselves. With tacit agreement, we are off!

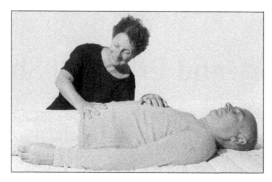

FIGURE 2.1: STILLNESS AND LISTENING

We know what Ki is

We are taught that Ki pervades everything, that everything is made of Ki. Though invisible in its purest form to most human eyes, it may be felt by clients and practitioners alike. As in all Shiatsu, Ki is what we are working with when we give a session to those who are facing death or who have experienced loss. Everyone sees the result of it, though they may not describe the origin of what they see in the same way that Shiatsu practitioners do. They see someone with tears in their eyes and a down-turned mouth and deduce from 'a feeling' that that person is sad. To a Shiatsu practitioner, sadness is a particular configuration and result of Ki. While the Metal energy is associated with breathing, and the direction of that element is said to be inwards and downwards, our clients pass through many subtle emotional changes and states, and each has variations (see Table 2.1) which those who read the body can observe.

Table 2.1: How Ki moves in the different states associated with death and loss

Stage	Breath	Direction	Location	Speed	State
Hope	Inhales and keeps on inhaling	Lifts, opens, forwards	Upper chest Crown chakra	Gentle	Brightening
Acceptance	Inhales, exhales, stops	Circles into centre	Hara and Heart Feet	Sits	Calm, integrated, grounded
Embarrassed	Holds	Folds over front inwards	Front, especially chest	Still, or very slow	Hiding
Denial	Holds	Back, in	Back of whole self	Slowish	Backing away, leaving a space
Anger	Staccato, short, exhales and inhales	Spreads out to sides Into Heart Opens	Throat, head, eyes, hands	Depends – can be sudden and immediate or slow and a gradual increasing in speed	Roaring
Realization	Slow inhale	Opens	Upper torso, all round, eyes widen	Quickish	Oh!
Disappointment	Exhales and keeps exhaling	In and down	Centre line, going through floor	Slowish	Sinks
Bargaining	Short inhalations	Forwards up from base chakra, sinking	Into hands, shin, upper body, heels, back arches	Constant moving	Pleading
Depression	Exhaling, very little	In and down	Solar plexus	Slow, stopped	Bleak, nothing
Relief	Air out of chest	Downwards	Torso	Quite quick	Release
Desperation	Inhale, inhale more, inhale more, hold	Pushing against eyes	Inside skin	Jammed up	Straining, taut

Cont.

Stage	Breath	Direction	Location	Speed	State
Resignation	Stopped after the exhalation	Inwards and downwards	Chest above diaphragm	Stiller	Collapsed, weak
Fear	Very little breath or quick short sharp inhalations	Backwards	Into head, throat, jaw, back of shoulders	Very slowly freezing	Retreating or frozen
The moment of shock	Sudden exhalation or inhalation	Scattered out from centre of chest	Out of and beyond the edges	Rush	Ah! (as of pain)
State of shock	Held	Scattered out from centre of chest	Out of and beyond the edges	Stopped	Arrested, blank
Panic	Small exhalations	Activity in chest All over the place	Drive from Kidneys	Quite quick	Wild
Dying	Comes and goes, stops, starts, 'rattle', periods of unconsciousness, space between them gets shorter	Interior	From the inside	Very slow, uneven	Slowing
Grief (thanks to Blanche Mulholland)	Compressed	In the whole body	Chest Closing of lower energetic centres In head in unconscious attempt to reconnect with deceased	Almost stopped	Compacted, amouring

In his book *No Death, No Fear*, Thich Nhat Hanh (2002, kindle edition) writes, 'The Buddha said that when conditions are sufficient something manifests and we say it exists. When one or two conditions fail and the thing does not manifest in the same way, we then say it does not exist.' Well, this is not far away from our beliefs about Ki. Thich Nhat Hanh goes on to say that we think a radio sound or television picture does not exist in the room if we cannot see it, despite knowing the radio waves are there all the time. It is of course the television and radio set which does not exist. As soon as they are in the room, there is the picture. It was the set which we needed to plug into the waves which then meant we could see the pictures – they were there all the time. The waves only seemed not to exist because we could not see them: 'the causes and conditions were not enough to make the television program manifest'.

At the end of life, clients can be receptive to energies which can connect them to phenomena that were previously inexplicable to them and this can confuse others around them. If someone has already lost consciousness, had a blood transfusion, if they are on certain drugs, they may have already had an experience. Similarly, someone who is grieving and has a sense of the spirit of the deceased being near, or seeing or hearing them, might be open for the first time to the existence of what we practitioners explain using the concept of Ki. Near death awareness recognizes that clients see those who have already died and have conversations with them when they are very close to death (Callanan and Kelley 2012).

Understanding Ki

In exactly the same way that we might not have understood Ki when we were starting to learn, so those who look through the eyes of science can struggle with the whole concept, and they may be the clients who are being referred to us at the end of life, or the very 'doorkeepers' of the places we need to be, the hospitals and hospices. The question is whether we will have to find ways to explain or demonstrate Ki if we want to share our work with those who are dying or grieving.

The Ki of the aim, diagnosis and results of a session

In general terms, we aim for a balance of Ki, working with the client's own sense of their Ki, engaging their self-awareness. If the client has died, the question of Ki balancing is quite different. The aim of this would be to support the Hun (see below, Traditional Chinese Medicine (TCM) and death). It depends on your own beliefs, but here you would be working with the spirit before it moves on and it is generally agreed that there is a very short time in which you can do this before the Ki ceases moving. Some practitioners have either instinctively continued to touch for a while, or wanted to and asked the client's Ki beforehand. It may be inappropriate, particularly if there are others present or if you have a strong sense that you do not want to touch for whatever reason.

Yin Yang

The theory of Yin and Yang, the first division from The One, the Tao, is our explanation of the way the world goes around. These concepts help us relate to our environment, giving us a point of reference. They are all about life, death and living harmoniously, encompassing one of the beauties of Chinese Medicine: simultaneous complexity and simplicity. Mutually arising and interdependent, all four principles tell us something about death and loss.

The circle (see Figure 2.2)

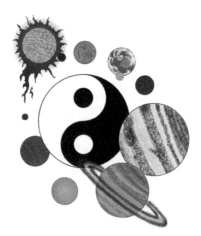

FIGURE 2.2: YIN YANG AND THE UNIVERSE

The circumference of continuous existence, ever moving and perfectly balanced, not only reassures in the purity of its singularity, but reminds us that we emanate from and are part of a whole – a cell, a community, a whole world and larger universe. It connects us with the cycles: the moon and the earth, the seasons, and our circadian rhythms of activity and sleep. On and on it goes, eternally flowing, a line which separates us from everything and everyone else. We are also contained within this membrane. As a symbol of never-ending Ki, we are reminded that we were, are, and will be. Being able to embody this explanation of existence as we enter the treatment or hospital room will centre us as practitioners, conferring a sense of clarity when we are with our clients who are enduring a time of chaos and distress.

The wholeness of the sphere is a reminder that every life, however truncated, is complete. Though we hear people speaking about lives cut short when someone dies at an early age, nevertheless each one has its own symmetry.

The curving line which divides the sphere

The wavy line which dissects the circle (see Figure 2.3) symbolizes the dynamic interplay between The Two, the surge and retreat of oppositional forces. As one is in the foreground, the other recedes; as pain surges there is less rest, then as pain lessens, relaxation increases. Active techniques such as rotations, alternated with quieter Tsubo work, mimic this ebb and flow of activity and stillness, thereby raising the client's awareness of it. Rocking, which causes waves literally to move through the body, will distract the client from her grief and, when it settles, may bring with it a realization that she can ride the fluctuating tides of life, that nothing will last forever.

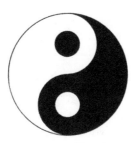

FIGURE 2.3: YIN YANG

Our ability to respond and react to change is encapsulated in the undulating line itself. As change happens, perhaps we are given some bad news, an impetus passes through us, a ripple or shock depending on the severity of the cause. The heartbeat gets raised, the breathing quickens – in short, the sympathetic nervous system prepares for fight or flight; later, it calms as the parasympathetic nervous system comes into play and we find a new balance.

The Water element, associated as it is with the autonomic nervous system, can be activated by sitting at the client's feet, gathering the ankles together close to the floor, and with the practitioner's Hara activating a side-to-side wave which transmits up the body to the head and back down again, finding the appropriate rhythm for that person's fluids.

Relative opposites

As two eyes in one face allow for focus and depth of vision, so too we must use both sides of ourselves to achieve balance and be able to see clearly, near and far. Our touch, for example, balances the Gallbladder meridian on the client's sides.

This can be done by standing up beside your client with your legs in a lunge. Hinge at the hips and place one palm on the right and the other on the left side of the client's body under their armpits. Keeping your knees and hips loose and initiating with your Hara, palm alternately in towards the centre line of their body, move downwards a little each time over the hips and down the legs. This will move their body slightly from side to side. Repeat. The third time, use both palms simultaneously so that there will be no sideways movement in the client.

This can help the two parts of the client focus together, perhaps recognizing how their past belief structures have connected with the current illness. If that does not improve their prognosis, they might be able to pass this knowing on to others.

Indivisible

A divided cell with a nucleus in each provides the potential for two sets of genes, two doses of intelligence (see Figure 2.4). We have two sides and they are equal, neither is more powerful nor weaker than the other. Neither can they be divided up; each exists because of its familiar and knows itself only by contrast and in comparison. There is not one thing which is without a counterpart, no 'only' without 'as well', and, so, no tragedy without deliverance. This is not to belittle a client's pain, but it is the law of nature that there will be a complementary side to it. If we can support our clients to metaphorically locate the conjoined sibling, perhaps by connecting the front and the back of the body in side position, they might find that life has a range of emotions and activities, both ill-health and wellbeing. Having these sides to life brings richness (though it is not always apparent at the time), and, indeed, wisdom that brings about the development of our species.

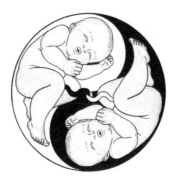

FIGURE 2.4: THE TWINS

Interdependent

Yin and Yang tell us that death is known because of life, that there is death in life, and imply that there is also life beyond death. Maybe we will be reborn, if not reincarnated, or perhaps our physical remains and energy will go to some use in the form of memories by loved ones or acts that continue to have an impact after the perpetrator of them has gone in body. Practitioners and clients alike may believe that there is nothing after we die – each one will make their own decision and Shiatsu can help provide mental space to consider this.

Transformation of Yin to Yang and Yang to Yin

Yin Yang tells us that an extreme of one transforms into the other. It could be argued that the more we appreciate living, the greater fear we have of death.

BF was a missionary, travelling overseas from England to proselytize. She never married, preferring to direct her prodigious energies towards those who needed aid. For 40 years, she moved among children in Africa and adults in Asia until her return to London where she shared a flat with many cats. As her spread of influence slowed, so her geographical location narrowed. When I first knew her she took a daily turn around the neighbourhood. A year later she rarely left her apartment, and six months after that she was almost chair-bound. She was chirpy and interested in the exploits of her nieces, nephews and helpers, and I was likewise drawn to make smaller movements and slow my pace as I gave her Shiatsu. While she had previously bemoaned her lack of adventure and flexibility, her awareness of what she enjoyed and what over-stretched her body helped her recognize her limitations and she ceased to push beyond them.

Yang had turned gently to Yin as BF's Jing decreased and the Shiatsu seemed to help her acknowledge that with dignity. Towards the end, she did not speak much, and whereas others in her vicinity could be heard to rant and rail through the walls, my client stayed calm. That could have been her personality, but maybe the Shiatsu assisted. The Yang of her Fire element had dulled, but the Yin still sparkled in her eyes when she saw me until the last few days of her life.

The theory is clear: if we are in tune with the Tao and live in the moment, conscious of each feeling and action, the greater the likelihood will be of our understanding the Way of All Things. Awareness of our humble and vital role in the universe will result in a deeper contribution to others, either as they are passing from one state to another, or managing the adjustment which will be the outcome of that death (see Figure 2.5).

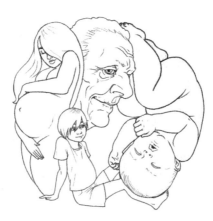

FIGURE 2.5: CYCLE OF LIFE

Trained to compare one thing to another and not deal with absolutes, to hold both the whole and its parts, to recognize the natural order of what is happening and to therefore let go of the need to be in control, we Shiatsu practitioners have something valuable to offer those who are grieving or at the end of life. If the entire session has activity as well as quiet, verbal engagement and silence, and hopes for a harmony between us and our client; if that is all related to their state on the day as well as the crisis or change of circumstances they are managing, then the holism of Yin Yang finds its manifestation in practice.

Traditional Chinese Medicine (TCM) and death

In our training, most of us were taught some TCM as background to and context for the bodywork; many have gone on to study and practise acupuncture in much greater detail. What follows is not a comprehensive account of TCM, only the parts which relate directly to death and loss. I am using the word Qi in this section, as it is the accepted version when writing about TCM.

The way I entered this theory was through the translations of the ancient texts and scholarly research of Giovanni Maciocia, Elisabeth Rochat de la Vallee and Claude Larre, Elizabeth Reninger and David Twicken (2004a). The majority of the information is about living a long and healthy life, as it should be, on being immortal even, but this does leave out the application to those who are dying. There is some instruction for 'calling back the soul to the body' (so someone can move on in peace), and bringing someone back from the dead, which I have not included because I have not tried it, have not found the need for it. So, armed with the jewels of information from the core texts, I worked practically in my clinic and on myself to arrive at what is below. It is useful to remember that, from the earliest beginnings, this 'theory' was developed experientially and it is therefore personal. While there are some commonalities, I encourage you to use it as a starting point for your own discovery, with yourself and your clients, in order to usefully embody it. I have offered some ways of exploring this in Chapter 7.

The information is relevant to Shiatsu practitioners who work in the area of death and loss because it elucidates some of the concerns and issues our clients express which are unexplained elsewhere. It is also the basis for most of our well-loved styles of Shiatsu, including the Five

Phases, Zen, and Movement Shiatsu, and therefore helps to understand them more fully.

Qi

Where there is Qi there is life; when it runs out, we die. Qi is the Oneness, the Source of universal life, and it lessens and abates at death.

The Po and the Hun

The Po and the Hun are the aspects of the soul which are concerned with death and loss. The Po is also closely allied to the Essence (Jing, fluids and so on), and the Hun to the Spirit (made up of the Shen, the Mind and more). According to Twicken (2004b) the focus of study is to understand the perpetual cycle of transformation, 'to harmonize these two influences or energies, obtaining health, balance and self-realization', and I would add, to have a good death.

The Po

The Po originates in the universal stream of Qi. At conception, it exits from there, is held in the mother's consciousness and her Blood, which together form the new life. According to tradition, the Po is more Yin and manifests with the first breath, but in my own experience it rides in on the mother's Blood and transfers to the baby via the bloodstream, thence to the breath and the Lungs. It is also called the Corporeal Soul, which has to be understood not as the physicality of the bodily entity, but as that which makes the physical animated. This name refers to where it goes at death. The Po is translated from the Chinese as the White (Body), which can be visualized as the mist of hot breath on a cold window or the whiteout of the Scottish haar. Its description by Maciocia (1989, p.139) as the 'somatic manifestation of the soul' speaks to me of its arrival into the body from the Universal Source.

Energetically, the Po arrives with a great rush of energy similar to a surfer riding a powerful wave. While with us, it bestows the consciousness of the breath, allowing dispersion, formation of borders, and communication. When it leaves it does not go quickly. As the gaps between the dying person's breaths lengthen, the Po which is surfing in the white foam of the breath stills for a time, then rides on, pauses and waits. (Remember that the Po and the breath are mutually enabling –

Maciocia (1989, p.139) calls breathing 'the pulsating of the Corporeal Soul'.) As the Po suspends, it recognizes, little by little, the change which is happening, that its carrier, the breath, has less and less energy. Then it suspends a last time. It is not a matter of the Po leaving now, but of it re-entering the stream of Qi, its function discharged. Traditionally, it then descends, down through the orifices (specifically the anus) into the earth, hence the name of Corporeal Soul. The Po is also more prosaically connected to mental inspiration and excreting the unwanted.

The Hun
The Hun is imparted to the baby by the father (Maciocia 1989, p.100), and is said to enter the body three days after birth. It is our connection to all Spirit. Imagine a stick of rock (the Qi) sliced through and showing the same pattern on both cut ends. That pattern is the pattern of the universal, the Hun, the part of me which is the same blueprint as everything else (not only human). It becomes supremely Yang after death and is known as the Ethereal Soul or Cloud (Body) as a result. Residing in the Liver, it is anchored by the Blood, but it is essentially independent, a slice of the universal which happens to be with us for our brief lifetime, connecting us with all things.

When our time comes, and if we have done what we should in accordance with the five instructions for a long life (quality food and drink, air, exercise, study and rest), the spirit of the Hun moves up and out into the air and shines in the Heavens. It is the way that our Qi lives on after we die, through the memories of others, the concrete work we do in our lifetime, the next incarnation, and through our progeny if we have them. The belief that the spirits of the dead remain part of the lives of the living is rooted in Buddhism. It maintains that link through taking care of the family grave and altar.

In life and after death
In life, the Hun and Po are a couple, 'two poles of the same phenomenon' (Maciocia 1989, p.124). Separate before birth, they come together during our lifespan, are stimulated and buoyed up by each other, and divide after death so we can 'have an afterlife' (Rochat de la Vallee and Larre 1995, p.42).

There are other aspects of TCM associated with death, as outlined below.

Essence (Jing) and the Kidneys

The Kidney function is related to the very cycle of life and to survival. It is concerned with the different stages of living – birth, puberty, menopause, old age – and death. In a simple way, the signs of ageing (thinning hair, a decline in hearing, weaker bones and so on) are an indication that this Organ and its Spirit, Jing – the vitality of this Essence – is dwindling. We are born with a certain amount of Jing and we can care for it so that it fades more slowly, but when it is used up, there is no more and we will die. The Kidneys are the outward expression of the Po, and also the way into it.

The Shen and the Chong Mai (Penetrating Vessel (PV))

The Chong Mai is the Sea of Blood and the Shen is the Heart spirit, one of the Treasures bestowed by the Hun. Picture yourself floating on the salty Aegean Sea, dreaming in the *shush* of it. That is like the Shen on the Sea of Blood. We saw, above, how closely associated the Blood is to the Po and the Hun. The presence of the Shen means we are recognizable as alive, whereas the Hun is beyond life and death.

The Shen and Blood as we are dying

As we are dying, the Shen is rescinded, revoked by the Hun to be restored to its former glory before the next time. In death, as the Shen tires, it is simply like a candle, it dims, and there is less and less shine. It darkens, blurs and extinguishes. At the same time, the Blood in the PV sea recedes, slowly drying up. (It is usually a result of a lack of fluids, although Heat from medical treatment and medication can hasten it.) With less oxygen, this Blood gets a darker red (a sort of eerie, Hallowe'en red version of the deep ocean or underwater cave where we can engage with the Kidney Qi), and it gets stickier. It is as if the dying person is listening to the ancient sound of the Blood, remembering being in the throbbing womb, remembering his ancestors who are in his Blood. His eyes are closed a lot of the time, he is deep inside himself preparing to go back from where he came. His Blood, however, is full of new memories and experiences from his life, which added to the ones from previous lives (however short his life was). Incrementally, he is starting to re-enter the slipstream of the Universal, via the Hun and the Po.

After death, the PV exists for a while because there is still Blood in the system, but as the latter is not illuminated by the Shen any longer, the sea also quite quickly dulls and becomes even more viscous. This means that there is no longer a job for the Hun, that the Ethereal Soul also has nothing to be lit up by, so it leaves, to merge with the Universal Spirit once more, and the ancestors.

Client fears explained through TCM

In the traditional theory of the Po and the Hun, you will find explanations for issues your clients may bring to you: fear of cemeteries and the dead; scary stories of spirits who have inhabited a living body; and fear of ghosts. These things are said to happen because someone either dies too young or has been violently killed, where 'the grasp of the Po' (Rochat de la Vallee and Larre 1995, p.41), being still strong, will not let go of life. Additionally, the ongoing bad luck of a client is said to be due to his ancestors who are haunting and taunting him, or not intervening with the Gods on his behalf. This causes havoc because the Hun is not being sufficiently honoured and appeased.

Blood transfusions

Like the sea, the Penetrating Vessel recedes when there is a crisis of Blood, a process of survival. Because of the relationship between the Hun, Shen and Blood, a blood transfusion brings with it another person or people's Qi, and it travels through the veins and into the Penetrating Vessel where the Qi of the Blood of the ancestors resides. There, it merges. This is a common procedure at the end of life and explains some people's experiences afterwards. It takes time for the newly introduced Blood to become integrated.

In conclusion, death is a gradual quietening of the Po before it enters once more into the Universal stream; the light of the Shen slowly dulls and is extinguished; the Blood in the PV gets darker and stickier so that it can no longer sustain the Hun, and so the Hun, the Ethereal Soul, returns to the spirits and ancestors.

The Five Elements

Note: I am assuming that the reader has a working knowledge and understanding of the basics of the Five Phases as I believe that all students learn this in their initial training. Please see the glossary if necessary.

Harriet Beinfeld wrote:

> The Chinese Medical vocabulary contained metaphors from nature like *Wood, Fire, Earth, Metal* and *Water, Heat, Wind* and *Cold*. This cosmological description of human process confirmed what I knew intuitively to be so – that what moves the world outside moves within me – that subject and object are two aspects of one phenomenal world. (Beinfeld and Korngold 1992, introduction)

Each of the Five Phases or Five Elements connects to death and related subjects with different associations, illuminating and directing us to ways in which we can help our clients. Some practitioners are skilled in identifying the client's constitutional or core element and are able to say that in essence this is an Earth (or Fire and so on) person. They know the archetypes and, after taking a case history and employing other forms of East Asian diagnosis, can identify the pattern of personality and habits. There is no one constitution which is associated with this book's topic.

Some are equally or more interested in the client's condition – an elemental state they can observe the person is passing through or stuck in for a while, one that is more significant at a given time. In any situation concerning grief, either when facing loss of life or if a loved one has died, it may well be a Metal phase of course. Whichever element comes to the fore, with attention it will be clear that the others are also present, and that there are periods when the client jumps back and forth between each of the five. Focusing on one or two in a session can be a lovely, simple way of working, and meeting the client like this can be a powerful acknowledgement of just where she is at that moment.

If there is a reason not to work one element directly because she is deluged by the symptoms associated with it, then the Shen (Creative or Mother and Child) and Ko (Control) cycles can be utilized (see Figure 2.6). They can address the key element through its *mother or controller* in the knowledge that this well-practised theory will provide what the client requires.

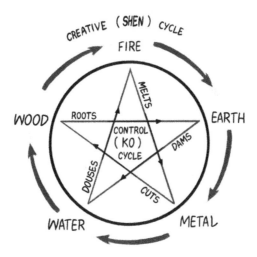

FIGURE 2.6: THE CYCLE OF THE FIVE ELEMENTS OR PHASES SHOWING
THE CREATIVE (SHEN) AND CONTROL (KO) RELATIONSHIPS

Alternatively, if the practitioner is working in the Zen way, the Five Phases can still be part of the session. The Conditional *element of the moment*, the one the client is most embodying on arrival, can be a theme for it: the two meridians from the Hara or back diagnosis will be worked, while also modelling and weaving that element throughout. For example, the client is in the first stage of shock after learning about the death of a friend in a car accident and the Fire element is uppermost. The Hara asks for Kidney Kyo and Stomach Jitsu, so the practitioner goes about her work, treating and balancing those two, while remembering that there has been a blow to the Heart and that therefore sensitivity and openness (qualities we associate with Fire) are particularly required in the session. It is likely that the two meridians presenting in the Hara are related to that element anyway: Kidney (Water) is in need of focus because the shock to Fire has evaporated it; Stomach (Earth), because Fire is no longer able to look after it on account of its need to self-focus, thus Earth is in danger of being neglected and unsupported.

Another manner of using the key element is to acknowledge it through the use of related techniques and body parts. In the example above, the practitioner decides to start with Kidney in the torso, but makes sure that when she gets to the upper part she adds in the Chest Centre (Tanzhong Conception Vessel or Ren 17, Heart Governor/Heart Protector/Pericardium Bo or Mu point) for dispersing any excess Ki;

perhaps also holding a listening palm over the centre of the chest to calm; and after working Kidney and Stomach in the arms, ensuring that a loving hand massage is given (the hands are closely related to the Fire element).

You can use also these techniques when working on yourself.

Metal

According to Pooley (2000, p.13), 'The Lung and the Large Intestine meridians integrate our concept of death.'

Metal is associated with grieving, sadness, loss and separation. Regarded as the first time period of the Chinese Clock, 3am–7am, it comes at a time of day when the bereaved may be lying awake missing a loved one and feeling alone.

The Metal element has an affinity with the season of autumn when nature lets go of the fruits of summer and the high season to prepare for winter. It is a time of year when those who dread the dark mornings and evenings (especially if they follow a 'traditional' work pattern and therefore rarely see daylight) can shrink into themselves. In response to the increased cold they can even move towards depression. The frail may wonder whether to give up and 'move on' at this time – the effects of the dying year are crystal clear and it seems a long time until spring. Despite the fact that much of the population is urban and disassociated with nature, the shortening of days and weather fluctuations nevertheless have a pronounced effect.

The Metal element has the ability to acknowledge the passing of all things, the *impermanence* as the Buddhists name it, to be in sorrow and express feelings about what has been. Using the diamond – a precious metal – as a metaphor, we see how paring things down to their innate structure can create a thing of beauty. All too often we resist this letting go process as we catch our breath, trying to keep contact with our dear ones who are no longer with us. The keening of a traditional funeral procession and the Heart's wailing tells us of the depth of putting asunder the realization that we are divided from the other. This fine exhalation clears the Lungs and makes way for the new breath.

Metal is, in fact, connected to the first breath a newborn takes after the cord has been cut or severed, marking the initial separation from the mother (in utero the foetus 'breathes' through the maternal blood). Mother and baby are no longer 'as one'. When the breath which began as we entered the world ceases, after the coming and going of the final stage of this incarnation, this apparently concrete existence is ended.

That first detachment and consequent independence from the mother marks the beginning. However, it is the father rather than the mother who is associated with this phase, and so the death of the patriarchal figure is even more significant if the client strongly identifies with this element. Gone is the archetypal disciplinarian, the one who says no and creates clear boundaries, and now is the time to integrate, or recognize that one has already integrated that function and will manage without the father, despite the obvious sadness. In addition, that client may already have had issues with the father before his death, complicating the response and suggesting that 'recovery' may be slow or that extra communication (psychotherapy, for example) is necessary. Should the grieving process prove too painful and outside support not be sought or be unavailable, depression can set in, withdrawal from society and loved ones can increase (as above), and the risk of taking one's own life grows.

For the client whose constitutional element is Metal, the releasing of the grief can be the sticking point.

TT (44 years old) struggled for breath after the short walk from the car. He had blue lips and the familiar barrel-chested appearance of someone with chronic obstructive pulmonary disease (COPD). He flopped down with a sigh followed by a cough. After a brief conversation, I slid a hand between the chair and his upper back and matched it with a palm in the centre of the chest. He began his story. In short sentences, he told me about the deterioration in his health, and how it got in the way of playing football with his second wife's teenage son. I repeated, 'Your second wife.' 'Yes,' he said, 'my first died in a car accident the December after we married, 12 and a half years ago.' There was a hiatus in conversation and breathing as I worked down the Lung meridian, focusing on Broken Sequence (Lie Que, Lung 7) in his left arm before holding his hand. He shut his eyes and I had the sense he was remembering. When he spoke again there was considerable emotion in his demeanour and he explained that although he was contented with his new relationship, he felt guilty because his previous spouse was so often on his mind.

The nurturing Earth, the Mother of Metal on the Creative or Shen cycle, with its fleshy touch and rocking and cradling, will help acknowledge the Yin of Metal (the empty hole of loss) if physical contact can be made. The balancing of the Fire element, however, utilizing the Control or Ko cycle, might help its Yang, which could be holding on to memories and not letting go of the tears and other emotions. Fire can also be used to melt the client's exterior borders, a psychological armour which was put on in an attempt to protect the self from the horror of living without. It must be noted that coping strategies such as these are or were present for a good reason and should therefore only be dismantled with the agreement of the client and with care.

Of course, the greatest gift to those in the Metal phase is breathing (pulmonary respiration), and while breathing exercises will help, they may also open the Lungs to the enormity of the loss and so are to be given with awareness. Perhaps they can be practised together in case they raise issues with the client, or maybe used in a holding exercise initially shared in silence.

Lying prone, PP, my client who had been recently bereaved and was now looking after her three children alone, was encouraged to concentrate on the breath as it moved in and out of her nostrils. Balancing on one knee and stepping forward on the other foot, I faced her head and started to palm down her back with both hands simultaneously. As she inhaled, I leaned forwards, meeting the top of her breath with my body weight; as she exhaled, I released and moved down a little. I followed her rhythm, changing pace if she took shorter or longer breaths, and repeating this until I reached the sacrum. She cried into the futon, and later, as we talked about her doing breathing exercises in the early hours of the morning when she found herself lying awake, she told me how alone she felt and admitted she needed help with the kids.

I am indebted to Audicia Morley for introducing me to this technique, and to Bill Palmer who taught me afterwards that bringing the client's attention to her expanded self also engages the Spleen function, making room for the Organs (the Lung pair in the Tai Yin) (Palmer 1996), which would explain why she became more aware of her needs as a mother.

Touch exercises like this one provide a gentle and safe way to focus on the client's breathing, while adding the support of the grounded and open-hearted practitioner. The Lung exercise of the Five Element Qi gong detailed in Chapter 8, Practical Exercises, can also be taught, as can a simple sitting and breathing meditation.

Earth

The Earth phase corresponds to the processes of understanding, the digestion of the reality of the loss. This is particularly connected to the mother, and her death will be a hard time for those identifiable as an Earth type, even more so as it will result in the breaking down or disturbance of the home and family unit.

Earth cradles and holds, croons while the sorrow racks the body. It offers sympathy, and accepts things simply as they are until they pass or change, until the bereaved can grasp their independence once more and move back into the world. When the client feels grounded and centred, perhaps as a result of the bodywork session, he knows that he will survive loss, understands that he is still connected to everything and can even give that opinion to others. If he can keep his feet on the earth he will continue to function, and the new information will be processed. If, however, he loses his footing and consequently his sense of stability, he might struggle to feel tethered and safe. The client can become bogged down in a mire of self-pity – not the healthy regard for self which results in extra care being given and support sought, but a state where he cannot move from the bed or sofa, is unable to care for his child or himself, and is in danger of becoming housebound. In this type of situation, touch almost always helps – the fleshy, nourishing sort of touch.

ZR's mother had died. Their relationship had been a painful mixture of separation and dependency, and now she was finding that the tension between needing support and an urge to cope alone was exacerbated. The grieving period had been a roller coaster of emotions in which she needed me to play a motherly role. I received desperate phone calls late at night and was accused of being unfeeling in sessions. Appointments were cancelled at the last minute. This is one sort of Earth element response to death.

The side effects of medication and Western medical treatment such as chemotherapy, which relate to the Earth phase, are nausea and a lack of appetite. Use of the Stomach meridian to descend the Ki, Ampuku Hara massage, and the Tsubos: Leg Three Mile (Zu san li, Stomach 36) and Central Stomach Exit (Ba hui, Ren 12, Stomach Bo point) usually helps.

Using the compassion of the Fire element, Mother to Earth on the Creative cycle, may mean that the under-nourished Earth client feels listened to, and the loving kindness of a friend, who perhaps knew the deceased from a distance, conveyed through social conversation, might be recommended. To engage the Control cycle, the Wood element is used: rooting, stretching and articulating through the Liver and Gallbladder meridians with more dynamic movement. The practitioner's plan here is to get the moribund client out of the quagmire and back onto solid ground.

Each time an aspect of the loss has been accepted and grounded (Earth), the client can move on into the transformation (Fire) stage.

Fire

The Fire element, which brings the warmth of the sun and of companions, can be extinguished by the fear of death, and can burn and consume when the client has lost control in the face of her own mortality. Faith can disappear, joy can be absent, and any sense of a connection to 'the bigger picture', the spiritual aspect of things, can be mere embers compared to the peace of mind before the grief had taken a hold. The ability to be calm and peaceful, sociable and to laugh, are things of the past – the spark has gone.

The shock of an unexpected death, particularly coming after previous ones, or of a beloved child, partner or pet, can even cause mental instability. In this case, the practitioner instinctively proffers a loving touch, meeting the client with compassion.

Hearing of terrible suffering caused by natural disasters, famine and war can set the Fire client's heart aflame with empathy. The Fire element must be settled before the client can find calm again. The client who usually exhibits a fine balance between meditation retreats and active networking finds himself reactive and emotional. In fact, he avoids walking to the village shop and takes the car, because meeting someone who shows kindness and asks how he is leaves him weeping on the pavement. Thus, he finds himself isolated and may regard the

Shiatsu practitioner as his new best friend. Kindly, we must maintain boundaries and can work the Fire meridians in towards the Heart. Paying tranquil attention to the back of the upper chest draws the Ki to the Heart centre, and holding the image in one's mind of a broken heart coming back into a whole helps focus on the session's aim.

The Mother of Fire on the Creative cycle is Wood, and this can be used as fuel. Engaging Wood's directness; putting the reality of the situation into words; viewing the soul's distress; and even using humour to lift the spirits are ways the practitioner could work. In addition, the insight of Wood can assist the client in seeing both sides of the situation, resulting in her ability to choose the right route where perhaps she must make a decision as to whether she can care for her mother at home or whether residential care is more suitable.

Working Bladder and Kidney in a flowing way, thereby using the Water element in the Control cycle, can metaphorically pour cool Water on a feverish body and mind, or maybe extinguish doubt and reconnect the receiver with her faith in God or a higher power, if appropriate for her.

KH had texted me in advance to arrange an emergency appointment as she had just returned from the hospital where she had been told she had breast cancer and needed immediate surgery. I knew her family history from previous sessions – her mother had died on the operating table from a heart attack during what should have been a simple procedure. She arrived in an agitated state, her arms flailing, her voice tone high pitched and her facial colour red. Within a few minutes of trying to explain her situation she started to have a panic attack. A panic attack involves extreme symptoms on various levels, and I deduced that KH was facing the possibility of death. I moved to the side of her as she sat on the mat, and placed a listening and firm hand on her shoulder. I palmed her back at a medium speed and said 'yes' in my mind, an affirmation for the Water element, a message to her system that it was managing well and would know what to do.

Water

The Water element, the ebb and flow of its emotions of courage and fear, is intrinsically connected with this book's subject. One way that clients face death is *with backbone*, that is, upright and with fortitude, and this is a facet of the Water element, as is seizing the courage to make life as fulfilling as possible in the knowledge that the end may come at any time. The right amount of stress, brought about by a particular diagnosis, for example, may motivate someone to make changes to diet, lifestyle or limiting belief structures which are needed to live the long life they desire.

Fear of danger protects from foolhardy behaviour, and nightmares can even serve to warn of serious problems that need to be addressed – both linked to the Water element. When out of balance, a cocksure, excessive sort of confidence takes your client up to the top of a mountain without the right gear. Alternatively, an overactive Water element might drown him in fear, immerse him in the horror of seemingly impending doom, or overwhelm with the sheer enormity of managing life after the loss of a partner through divorce.

When fear is the stage of grief that your client cannot move on from, the Water element is uppermost. Unable to let his child go to school alone after a neighbour's child was run over on the way there, he is restricted to going to work late and his stress levels build. Not only that, but he finds himself crying out a warning if he sees a toddler running down towards a crossing even when adults are around for safety. Arriving at the office shaking, he becomes increasingly unable to take decisions and that is what brings him to Shiatsu. Receiving flowing sessions in a structured manner slowly restores his equanimity.

Sitting back-to-back with your client can help to assuage apprehension: invite them to lean against you, giving you their body weight. If they have the energy, they can raise their hips and tip further backwards towards you, so that you are folded forwards over your thighs in the Water Makko-ho stretch and their spine is opening while being fully supported by your back. This is a dual Bladder meridian workout. Note that the second part might be too strong in certain circumstances, so, if you are unfamiliar with it, try with a friend first. Then, knowing how it feels for you, you can make the right choice for your clients.

The sensible guidelines of Metal (Mother of Water), and the containment that could be put in place by using the Lung and Large Intestine meridians, are a way of using the Creative cycle. The lifeline which is the prerogative of a centred Earth touch, that is, using Water's Controller, or the reassurance of a motherly foot massage, could be helpful in damming that flood and calming the tidal wave.

Premature ageing can be the result of chemotherapy or hormone treatment – early menopause, hair falling out, ear problems, dryness, sleep problems – but learning to take things at a wholly different pace and engaging the acceptance of the Earth element might lessen these effects.

Wood

The emotion associated with Wood is anger, and that often plays a part in people's attitude to death; indeed, it is the second of Elisabeth Kübler-Ross's 'Five Stages of Grief' (Kübler-Ross and Kessler 2005). It is usually a result of feeling out of control, of knowing that we cannot always choose.

Tiziano Terzani (2004) retells an old Indian tale in his *One More Ride on the Merry-Go-Round* of a man who is sent by his master to a bazaar for food. While there he sees Death in her grey robes (it is a female personification in his version) and gets a fright. He rushes back to the house and begs for a horse so he may escape. His boss complies and off rides the servant at top speed to Samarkand to get away. The Master is intrigued and makes a trip of his own to the bazaar. There he finds Death and berates her, 'Why did you scare my servant?' She replies that she was most surprised at the servant's behaviour towards her, saying that he had had no need to fear. 'Our meeting,' she adds, sending a chill up my spine as I read it, 'is tonight in Samarkand.'

This is a story, but the truth is that we all know people who were healthy and did not smoke, or 'so young with everything in front of them' to whom Death came anyway.

Anger and rage may lodge, stagnate and be therefore very slow in moving. It can be directed towards the deceased as well as the survivors, towards those who are lucky enough to still have their mother or best friend alive, or indeed at the whole world. Those who are desperately trying to negotiate a new reality after death and come to terms with what might have been an unbelievable and terrible accident scream, 'Why did I not know it would be like this?' (see Jayson Greene's *Once More We Saw Stars* (2019), in which his daughter was out with her grandmother and a brick fell on her, from which she never recovered.)

There are many other reasons why anger comes to the fore at a time when you might have thought your client would be simply sad. For example, perhaps the treatment given was erroneous. A client who was already on medication was prescribed a second one by a general practitioner (GP) and they clashed with devastating effect. The pharmacist at the hospital also failed to notice. She nearly died and was left with severe issues. There are countless reasons why anger can be at the forefront as the grief process plays out, including directing it at the deceased person themselves, feeling deserted by them.

Although there are Chinese Medical tomes promising a long life, implying that if you do x, y and z you will live into old age, most of us do not know when we will die. It is this lack of ability to see into the future, to choose the way and time of going, that can result in frustration and sometimes this is directed at the practitioner. Of course, it is not we who caused it, but we can help the client to recognize this and perhaps even forgive themselves or others who were involved.

Clients, in fact all of us, are prone to bargain or be incredulous if faced with death: 'But I am good,' we say. 'If I work hard, keep healthy and follow the rules, surely I deserve to be spared, to have a long life?' We barter and offer an exchange, 'my life for my daughter's', and the disappointment and anger we might feel when this does not materialize injures the Wood element.

Our clients may find that making the next small choice towards life, or, if unwell, towards a better death, can cause difficulty if we have developed or inherited habits which get in the way of this decision making. The Wood element is associated with addiction, particularly to alcohol and drugs (over-the-counter or illegal), and to work, danger and more. We might ask if this is a way our clients choose to forget about, to avoid, or to hasten their death. To answer those questions, we need of course to listen to each individual. Because the behaviour is not the underlying cause, we must listen to each individual, and using a Wood technique such as straight talking may uncover what lies beneath.

The Liver is associated with the Wood element and physiologically deals with metabolizing toxins. Chemotherapy is the most serious group of poisons we are knowingly prescribed. (Human Immunodeficiency Virus (HIV) medication is similar, but nowadays it is given more gradually than some of the aggressive chemotherapy treatments.) The pressure on that organ will be enormous and the response will depend on its former health and the lifestyle followed, both at the same time as treatment and afterwards.

When met with a serious diagnosis, the client may only have a short time in which to make a decision (this is the reign of the Gallbladder, of course). If the decision is to undergo treatment, then it can be followed by heavy medications. Accompanying debilitation means that exercise is exhausting and the body weak, but lack of movement means that the Ki can easily stagnate, something which additionally puts a strain on the liver. What a burden for the largest organ of the human body!

What to do? Liberating the joints and their attachments, the muscles, tendons and ligaments, engages the Wood element. A direct touch and other techniques which move the Ki might be appropriate where the client is strong enough. With a weaker patient, who is atrophied or stiff from prolonged bedrest, micro-rotations may be more suitable.

> Micro-rotations start from a place of health or ease within the receiver's system. Working within the boundary of movement which is safe for the client, we use very small movements, sometimes almost imperceptible to the eye. Starting by locating a centre point for rotation (may be Tsubo), they are performed gently and usually slowly and it is important to support with a two-handed contact. We work with breath to aid opening and relaxation in the area, 'taking up the slack' then stretching, and listening to the body's response. Intention is crucial and visualizations can be helpful (expanding and spiralling motions). Feedback from the receiver and respecting the boundaries of movement are very important. (Jill Fraser)[1]

The client usually knows what feels right in the Shiatsu session, although in the case of someone with strong Wood tendencies, they may expect more than is really possible or want to challenge themselves. In this case, the practitioner must follow her intuition and be creative, knowing that less and gentler work may be best, but it could release any anger lying under the surface and so it is good to have ways to manage that. Clean Language (Pole 2017) is ideal as it allows the client to hear their own words, to have a second chance to listen to what is going on in the bodymind, and to engage the right hemisphere's innate understanding (a different sort of knowledge from the left hemisphere's logical approach).

To be in a balanced relationship with your client who is often showing Woody signs, or who is in a Wood Phase just now, is vital. Noticing his relational habits and your own behaviour when you are with him will give you a clue. Do you feel defensive? Do you feel

---

1   Jill Fraser (2012) *Micro-rotations handout/TSSED/12/06/2012* page 2.

defeated, powerful or pathetic? Spend some time reflecting back to him. Taking it to your supervision session so that you are working on his case with someone else will draw attention to the push and pull between you. Ask yourself, who is the bulldozer and who the doormat; that is, who pushes on regardless of other people or internal feelings, and who finds himself constantly standing back and letting others or feelings overpower him? The answer could be useful for the client who is frustrated by a prolonged hospital stay, or is unable to work or be with the family she loves.

Working without the need for words in an active and harmonious relationship where you can use pushing and yielding on both sides will mobilize the Yin and Yang of Wood. It could be that the practitioner moves the body and the client allows that; or that the client insists on a strategy and the practitioner goes along with it. Working in either way, or preferably with a mixture of the two, will engage the client who is in a Wood phase. It is important that the client can practise choice-making in a safe place where, if it results in an outburst or collapse of indecision, the situation can be acknowledged and perhaps protocols found to support for the future.

Being able to make plans or not being able to 'see into the distance' is a feature of a Wood pattern. Faced with his mortality, your client may not be able to see beyond the fact that he might die today. Directly naming this, either wordlessly through mindful bodywork or in conversation, a plan to make that bucket list and follow it through can help. It is possible, though, that it may go in the other direction, into inaction followed by depression and withdrawal, in which case the Ki is backing up along the Control cycle and the Metal element is the new Condition. (Note that, in TCM, depression is a recognized facet of Wood, not Metal.)

Using the Creative cycle, Water is the *mother* of Wood, and working with that element will perhaps bring flow where Ki is stuck. The intention in using the Metal element, the Controller of Wood, might be to lay down some rules (restricting alcohol intake to two glasses per day, for example), or to let go of unhelpful emotions and to encourage deeper breathing to make space between angry outpourings (both these latter behaviour patterns are commonly met in nursing homes for the elderly).

In conclusion, the theory and practice of the Five Phases or Five Elements has a lot to offer the practitioner who is working with clients facing or dealing with death. They provide a method of diagnosis as well as ideas for treatment and recommendations, and are an ideal way to approach sessions which may be emotionally and spiritually highly charged.

Zen Shiatsu

Pauline Sasaki and Cliff Andrews have pioneered The Four Levels of Zen Shiatsu and Quantum Shiatsu in the UK and the rest of Europe (see Table 2.2), and much of the content in this section is inspired by them and other teachers who trained or worked alongside Sasaki. This section assumes understanding of the basic concepts of, and relationship between, Kyo and Jitsu. For an explanation of this, please see *Shiatsu Theory and Practice* (Beresford-Cooke 2011, p.146).

Table 2.2: The Four Levels of Zen Shiatsu with related information

Level	Physical	Emotional	Mental	Spiritual
Associated with	Pain, other symptoms associated with life-threatening illness or dying such as bowel, bladder issues; surgery; hair falling out; immune system stress; eating, drinking and breathing issues; resuscitation and being kept alive, coma.	Feelings: sadness, fear, anger, happiness, shame. State of mind: melancholy, longing, missing, wishing, horror, shock, frustration.	Thoughts, decisions, worry.	Connection with religion (God, Allah, Yahweh), nature, other people, animals, birds, insects, angels, Gods and goddesses, enlightenment, dreaming.
Questions	What will happen to my body now? Will I suffer? Will I be in pain? Will I be able to breathe?	What will happen to me now? Will I be brave or scared?	What will happen to me now? Where will I go? How will my relatives cope? What about my clients? What if I made a mistake?	What will happen to me now? How will I go on? What is the point? Will anyone remember me? Was it worth it? Did I make a difference? Did I do or say enough?

Cont.

Level	Physical	Emotional	Mental	Spiritual
Fear	Of pain, of losing my mind.	Of losing control of my emotions.	Of death.	Of heaven, hell or nothingness.
Decisions	To accept pain relief.	To accept that I cannot cope, to accept help.	To be buried, to stop treatment, to commit suicide, to stop work.	To give up, to trust that all will be well.

In Zen Shiatsu, we work with what is happening now, in the moment; the Hara diagnosis reveals a snapshot of the client's Ki at the time we touch and engage with it. For those in pain, panic or mental anguish, in a coma or dying, this way of working is ideal. There is less need to look at past patterns because the current situation is calling out for attention, and acute situations at the end of life call for shorter treatments. If the sessions are shorter or energy levels (of the client or practitioner) are reduced, if there is some sort of emergency, Zen Shiatsu is highly appropriate. Communicating with the client like this makes for a simple and quick connection, and causes minimal disturbance.

All Ki moves at a frequency, and human vibrations vary according to situation, temperature, mood and so on. The rate of vibration, which constitutes a wave in the electro-magnetic field of the human system and the air around it, is what we are tuning in to or picking up when we do Shiatsu. Whereas the practitioner's wave and the client's wave are likely to be vibrating differently before meeting, when the contact is satisfying and the connection effective, these waves flow together. Empathy relies on this connection, and compassion and sympathy are the results of it. Sharing feelings or thoughts, knowing instinctively where to touch and how, are signs that the frequency of the practitioner and client is closely related. Moreover, depending on what zone we are in – feeling (grieving, for example), thinking (worrying about how the children will manage), physically being aware of a bodily sensation, or being at one with the spirit that made us, our frequency changes. It is the particular skill of the Shiatsu practitioner to not only be able to align and harmonize with a client's frequency, but also to know that is happening and be able to respond accordingly.

ED was in a supine position on the massage table. She was breathing extra heavily, which could have been the exertion of walking to the treatment room, as well as her lung cancer. She was lying in a very stiff, uncomfortable-looking way. She just shook her head when I asked her how she was. I started with a Hara diagnosis and asked her whether she would like me to touch her legs or not. Thumbs up! I left one hand on her Hara and slid the other under her thigh, starting to lever up as I worked along the Large Intestine meridian (Large Intestine was Kyo in the Hara diagnosis). She winced. I slowed down, waiting longer at each point than usual and she started to relax. By the time I got to her foot for the first time she had shut her eyes: we had started to harmonize. Afterwards, I worked the Stomach meridian (which was Jitsu in the Hara) in a similar way, and that was when she started to tell me her story.

Finding and working the Kyo which is related to the painful place

Holding or having the palm of the Mother hand on the painful location, the Jitsu (because it is the known aspect, and it calls attention to itself), and exploring with the active hand along the same meridian, allows you to identify the Kyo places which belong to that Jitsu and may relieve it. There may be one or more Kyo area that is connected to the pain and each will have an energetic link which you can harmonize for the sake of greater integration of the bodymind.

SL was experiencing lower pelvic pain (4 on a scale of 1 to 5 where 1 is low and 5 is high) after a hysterectomy, and although she wanted to lie on the floor, she winced as she got down. The area was swollen and inflamed internally, she reported, and the discomfort interrupted her sleep. Rather than wanting me to avoid the area, she asked me to touch, but deep thumbing was obviously impossible on that day. I explained that my intention was to address the pain via other connected places to see if it brought any relief and she agreed. Placing my Mother hand slowly there and engaging energetically with the place where the uterus had been, I moved her leg into the Spleen stretch position and started to palm up the Spleen meridian (from Spleen 1–11) on that side, leaving my hand in each place for several seconds and noting the feedback under my Mother hand. When I found a site where there was a reaction I switched to thumbing with the active hand and we worked together, identifying the right depth and length of stay. I performed basic foot Shiatsu before repeating on the other side, and this was enough for her energy levels. She got up without pain and reported reduced levels (1–2) at the next session.

Modelling the meridian functions and giving recommendations

Cliff Andrews (2012, p.4) writes, 'The Kyo and Jitsu Meridians can be experienced as two dominant qualities, or movements or vibrations, which contribute to the overall way that the Ki field is expressing itself.' We can use the Kyo meridian functions to guide us throughout a session with those facing death, and to offer a suggestion to the client for prolonging its benefit and supporting themselves afterwards. For example, if a client had recently received a terminal diagnosis, appeared to be scared and the Hara diagnosis was Kidney Kyo, Small Intestine Jitsu, we might choose to work at the emotional level for shock and fear. Engaging with our own fear of death as we work, we do not speak about it, or attempt to influence the client, neither do we become overwhelmed by it, but we interact with it internally, knowing that the Ki field will be affected. Being congruent with our fear will affect our own vibration and bring us into resonance with the client.

If the client then seeks a recommendation, we can base it on the composite of the Kyo and Jitsu and, in the example above, recommend a hot water bottle for the kidneys.

Do not assume that because the client is at the end of their life, the spiritual level is always the best way to address his Ki. Pauline Sasaki (2001) writes:

A receiver who has no CONSCIOUS concept of energy will tend not to feel what you are doing off of the body and therefore not respond. Of course, on an unconscious level, you may feel a lot happening to the receiver energetically, but it will not connect up consciously with the receiver, so they may feel nothing has happened…a person with a low kinaesthetic sense is very much in touch with the slower, denser vibrational energy. This range of vibration includes the vibrational range of the human form. Therefore, if you work on the body, it is very easy for the receiver to sense what you are doing and assist you in creating energetic changes.

Zen Shiatsu and grief

Working with clients using Zen Shiatsu usually involves working from a back or Hara diagnosis, even if the practitioner knows that grief is the primary symptom. There are meridian functions which theoretically pertain to certain aspects of grief, and in the absence of a diagnosis these can be used as a starting point. However, you will see from Table 3.2 that all the meridians can be connected, so begin there to give you time to settle into yourself, then follow the Ki.

Techniques inspired by Movement Shiatsu

I do not describe myself as a Movement Shiatsu practitioner, but have been using some of the concepts, techniques and experiential anatomy in my work since 1992. Learned, in most part, from Bill Palmer or Audicia Morley, they are embedded in my Shiatsu, such that my hands automatically conjure them when the situation arises.

The role of the client

Perhaps one of the most inspiring things is that the client knows what she needs and is already exhibiting it in her movements, striving towards wholeness as we all are. I have found this attitude to be extremely useful when giving Shiatsu to those who are grieving or dying and at times of crisis. When there are no words to describe what is needed or when it is impossible to utter any; where the body has become almost completely paralysed; then the ability to identify even a spark of a gesture or semblance of an action gives me somewhere to start and is invaluable. Noticing it, mirroring and gently amplifying it, supporting it in its journey to fulfilment, takes the client to surprising and often deeply satisfying places. It sometimes even seems to complete something which started in the womb or shortly after birth, but has never before reached its dénouement.

Valuing the Jitsu

In Zen Shiatsu, there is a dynamic interplay between Kyo and Jitsu, akin to that of Yin and Yang, but more so: Kyo is the cause of Jitsu and so is very often treated first. Once this hidden or unexpressed causal Ki is met and acknowledged, so Shizuto Masunaga's theory goes, the Jitsu will be able to release from its role of signpost for, and expression of, the Kyo, and any straining or excessive behaviour can then be released – a new balance has been found. However, after defining the two terms in a paper he wrote on the subject, Palmer (2013, p.2) argues that there are times when the Jitsu must be addressed immediately, and nowhere is this more apparent than in end-of-life care or when someone is in distress. Time is of the essence and matters are pressing. The practitioner starts, instead, with the most obvious, listening to the part with the loudest voice. Only when that has no need to shout as loudly any more does the practitioner then turn his attention to the underlying quieter one. Palmer (2013, p2). wrote, 'If you start working with a place that is already alive and embodied, then this empowers them [the client] and they have the confidence to go with you into the problematic parts.'

Proximal–Distal and taking up the slack

(Of the two bones which meet at a joint, the proximal is that which is closest to the Hara, and the distal is the one which is at the furthest distance from it.)

Using the Proximal–Distal technique with my client, I am looking for equal movement of the proximal and distal bones which make up a joint. My aim is for the body to move more sequentially (from the centre out to the extremities). This brings a gentle softness to the articulation which is soothing to those who are either unable to move themselves or where oedema, for example, has brought the body to a veritable standstill.

Cynthia Shuken (2013, p.1) writes:

'Taking up the slack' is about making a connection, either with another person or within yourself. If our touch is too lax, we (and the other) cannot really feel any connection; if it is too firm or tight, it doesn't allow for movement. This is very important when we are contacting the meridian or Tsubo – our pressure needs to be firm enough that we both feel a connection, but not so much pressure that we stop or impede the movement of Ki. If we are doing a stretch on a partner, having firm enough tension means we can feel what is happening in a muscle, bone or joint. If our tension is too loose, neither we nor the client can feel much, and the stretch is ineffective. If it is too tight, we cannot feel much, either, as there is no room for movement (there can even be increased resistance, which impedes movement further).

'Taking up the slack' is another technique that can be used in an internal, subtle way with a bedridden client who is struggling for autonomy of movement. It can introduce the subtlest Eccentric Contraction (the tone a muscle has while lengthening), and promote awareness of tensegrity (the elastic connection holding everything together). This is a movement of energy, motivating the Ki and connecting up body parts.

Palmer (2019) writes:

> I find the concept of Taking up the Slack really useful in extreme old age, as with the Proximal–Distal work…however, the concept of Valuing Touch, touching a tense muscle in a way that it can feel you are not trying to make it let go and are valuing its contribution, I have found really helpful at that last stage of life.

Other Shiatsu styles

When working with clients at the end of life, or in distress, especially spiritual distress, the practical techniques will be useful. Katharine Hall (2010, pp.6–8) wrote about what she does in mental health institutions:

> How most usefully to work? Tongue diagnosis and then meridian and point work? Hara and meridian work and grounding, spirit support? East Asian interpretation of client's energy state and ideas for supporting the self outside of sessions? My work usually includes a combination of these… Shiatsu Practitioners' professional training with its range of theory and practical skills taught, and the self-reflection required, are excellent grounding… I believe practitioners offer real benefits to the NHS (UK National Health Service) as well.

Integrating non-Shiatsu modalities

The practitioner may also find that other modalities of touch, or working with sound, colour, crystals and poetry, simply happen when working at the end of life. Counselling skills, Reiki or Shamanism, prayers and so on, even if not employed in everyday practice, have featured regularly when I have asked my colleagues how they work in these circumstances.

Sotai

Sotai (Dr Keizo Hashimoto's technique of postural realignment) is 'based on the principle of regaining health through natural pain free movement' (Liechti 2004/2012[2]). This is ideal for working with those in the throes of grief, as their system is already overloaded. A system where the practitioner goes to the place of ease, and in the direction of least resistance, rather than challenging the client, can be highly suitable.

Seiki

Seiki (see the writing and teaching of Alice Whieldon after her work with Akinobu Kishi, 2011, p.92) is realized through contact called 'life resonance' which, in recognizing that 'a patient becomes open and shows me', acknowledges the powerful participation of the client. This way of working is infinitely connected and responsive, ideal with the seriously sick or frail.

Working with the Light Bodies and Light Body Activation

Some Shiatsu practitioners call on the aid of higher beings, deceased relatives or guardians of the client. This may connect with what are more frequently referred to as Light Bodies (auras), and other, even more expansive energies if your client is at the end of their life or facing their inevitable death. However soon that comes around, the client's spiritual self is already primed for this type of work if they are near the end of life.

Gabriela Poli describes Light Body Activation, Shiatsu which specifically engages the light body, as 'high vibrations [which] influence

---

2   From a handout supplied during a workshop.

the physical tissues',[3] and so, once again, this is appropriate with those facing death and loss.

Chakras

The suggested instructions below refer to the chakras – seven spiralling vortexes of energy along the central line of the human body, which together make up their own system and are part of the Indian Ayurvedic tradition. Four of the chakras are listed here as they are particularly connected with death and loss.

The base chakra

Located in the area of Long Strong (Chang qiang, GV or Du 1) and Meeting of Yin (Huiyin, CV or Ren 1) and encompassing the Ki of the beginnings of these two central and Extraordinary channels. The base chakra connects with the earth. For those facing life without a loved one, the base chakra keeps their feet on the ground when all around them has changed – somewhere to refer and come back to.

The heart chakra

Located in the middle of the chest, between and encompassing the acupoints Chest Centre (Dan zhong, CV or Ren 17, the HG Bo or Mu point) on the front of the body, and the HG Yu point (Jue yin shu, BL 14) and the HT Yu point (Xin shu, BL 15) on the back. The heart chakra connects with the energy of the Heart. As a client with a terminal diagnosis prepares to leave her family, her heart chakra will open and flood with both love and pain.

> Our hearts feel passion, the effects of suffering, as well as love. The love and the pain can be very difficult to separate, but when we can allow ourselves to feel both, we see that the pain can shift and it can change. When we allow Anahata [the heart chakra] to open to all the qualities it holds, we understand that they can exist together: in love, and in pain. (Helbert 2019, p.145)

---

3   Gabriela Poli in a New Energy Body webinar about light body work perpetuated by her with Nicola Pooley after the death of Pauline Sasaki.

The third eye chakra

Located between the eyebrows in the region of the Extra Point, *yin tang* and between there and Mute's Gate (Ya men, GV or Du 15) and Wind Mansion (Feng fu, GV or Du 16) plus Celestial Pillar (Tian zhu, BL 10). Also related to the upper Dantian. The third eye chakra connects with the intuition and the mind, and will support a client in finding peace when they are facing death or coping with loss.

The crown chakra

Located around the uppermost acupoint of the human body, and closely related to Place of 100 Meetings (Bai hui, GV or Du 20). The crown chakra is the doorway between the body and the heavens and connects with the universe in its enormity and breadth. Release from suffering, connection with other realms and the Subtle Bodies are connected with the crown chakra.

Other

Treating one body part through another

The body is a series of parts linked by fascia. The fascia wraps around the organs, muscular structures, channels and so on, intricately attaching one to the other like double-sided sticky tape. This facilitating of energy exchange and communication – transmitting through their sinuous pathways – goes some way to explaining how we can treat one part of the body with and through another, when the first is unable to be touched. At the end of life, when physical pressure is uncomfortable or injurious in certain areas (perhaps a scar from recent surgery or the site of radiotherapy), this technique can be used. I have used some valuable metaphors which I first heard in a workshop given by Wilfried Rappenecker in 2017.

A client has pain in his right and left feet, ankles and legs from severe oedema. I see that they are red and swollen and feel the heat emanating from them without touching. He cannot sleep or bear even the touch of light bedcovers. I take the hand which he holds out to me.

1. I try to *sit comfortably in his hand, as if in an armchair*, using a relaxed and open attention.

2. I am interested in how I feel, and what his hand is like: the skin, the flesh and bones, the temperature, weight, whether more Yin or Yang, Kyo or Jitsu. I note what arises on all levels.

3. Maintaining my focused attention, *I imagine that I have a fishing rod in my hand and cast the line out and down his body to his legs* and focus there for a while, seeing what arises.

4. Moving, then, between the hand which I am holding and the part I have *landed* on, I focus on the connection between them.

5. I remind myself that the client's aim is relief from the pain and sensitivity in his legs, and know that my intention is to give hand Shiatsu for that reason.

6. When the time is up, I withdraw my attention from the legs, back to his hand, and focus there, once more, noting any changes.

7. After silently thanking him, I pay attention to myself and then replace his hand on the bed.

Number 1 above, being comfortable, is important for establishing resonance, which Wilfried Rappenecker (2001, p.2) succinctly described as a 'reciprocal vibration. It means understanding a shared experience.'

What you can do when you do not know what to do

When faced with situations which are upsetting or complicated, it can be hard to be centred enough to make a diagnosis. Here is a general list which includes a mixture of techniques from different modalities, to get you started:

- I was introduced to this technique by Pauline Sasaki and have used it many times (and may have unwittingly changed it, since it was a long while ago). Sitting still and quietly, let your hand rest on your client's Hara. Make a good connection. Tune in. Imagine two speech bubbles above your head: the first has Kyo written in it and the second has Jitsu. Both also have space in them. Now silently ask, which is the Kyo meridian? See it appear in the space under the word Kyo in the first bubble. Do the same for the Jitsu. Go right ahead and work those two.

- Think of what the client has told you and work the elements, points or meridian(s) which jump into your mind. In the absence of words, use your own sense of which ones feel right and trust that your Ki does know, even if your mind does not recognize that.

- If you can identify a clear symptom, for example the client is breathing very fast, use the element, or a meridian or technique, which is associated with that. In this case, start by touching their Hara or another accessible part, and do practise some deep belly breathing. See what happens next.

Working on a table or hospital bed

When working with grieving relatives in a hospice, you may be working in a small therapy room with no futon, only a massage table. If giving Shiatsu in the hospital, you may be limited to a hospital bed which has a squashy mattress, side and end bars (though they may be removable) and table and chairs all around it. Additionally, the client could be attached to a feeding tube, an oxygen line and other paraphernalia restricting your access.

Massage table

Most modern massage tables have adjustable height and end sections. The client may need his head raised if there are breathing difficulties, and his feet if oedema or other circulatory issues are present. For your own comfort and ability to reach and execute the Shiatsu you choose, experiment with finding the right arrangement: for example, you might like the table to be low down, if it has that capacity, so that you can lean your bodyweight down – as long as you return it to a 'normal' level for the client to dismount, that should work well. The focus, as ever, is to connect with the Ki. Jane Groombridge (2019) has been working on a table for years and says: 'I have a stronger sense of a different dimension of energy around the table than on the floor.'

Hospital bed

If your client is comfortable with the idea, you could get onto the bed with him to achieve the closeness you are used to on the futon. (Check it is strong enough first!) Otherwise, depending on your height, you will have to be very careful about your back. Regular yoga practice and other strengthening activities will support you in this. Even if you are a volunteer, you can often get patient-handling and safety courses for free from those who are familiar with hospital equipment (think of them as payment in kind, as they will benefit all of your practice).

Grounding

As Andrew Staib (2019) stressed in his workshop given at the Shiatsu Society Congress, grounding yourself cannot be overestimated:

> Using the support from the earth and going down in the legs, the Ki rises back up and out through your hands. Use your heels to anchor the whole body and your big toes for support when you lean forward with diagonal alignment. Notice how your centre of gravity becomes very low in the body. Your Hara should be positioned between your knees, as in the horseriding stance, and it is important that the deep core abdominal muscles are activated, especially on the outbreath. Activating Kidney 1 will enliven the whole Kidney meridian, right up into the chest, allowing the spine to feel straight and naturally supported.

As with futon Shiatsu, Staib (2019) added, 'I am actually gently using the client's body as "support" as I lean in, and then feeling their body's life energy pushing back to me.'

Comparison with the futon

There are aspects of giving Shiatsu which are easier on a table, and elbows and forearms are very useful adjuncts if you do not always use them. Jane Groombridge (2019) writes:

> You can gain better access for working around the neck in supine, and the back in side position. Wider movements are possible with arm stretches, and with a handy stool you can sit to work the feet, which avoids stooping. It is more familiar to some folk because they are consulted on a table when they visit the doctor, physiotherapist or osteopath. However, it is less grounded than being on the floor with the practitioner's bodyweight above them.

Contraindications

When working with someone at the end of life, the contraindications which we use for the rest of our work and which apply to so many clients can be obsolete. The medical focus at this stage is usually on pain relief and symptom control to enable the patient to live as fully as possible until she dies. Working as part of a complementary healthcare team, you may also be expected to focus on those things. In the day clinic, referrals may come from the physiotherapist or occupational therapist and therefore may be practical, to do with ambulation, side effects such as oedema, older symptoms such as arthritis, or practical support for a wheelchair user who has stiffness in the hips or sore shoulders from manoeuvring the vehicle. There may also be a counsellor and spiritual adviser or chaplain present in your workplace which may preclude or obviate the need for you to address the emotional or spiritual aspects. Or it may not – we know how much Shiatsu offers and that any physical work will have an effect on the entire bodymind. I respect the other professionals working with my clients and I follow my intuition. It is hard to change what we do and it is also inappropriate. Being expected to work on a purely physical level shows a lack of understanding from mainstream health staff, and thus we seek to further educate them about our profession.

Recent surgery

We teach students not to give Shiatsu after recent surgery, the amount of time varying from a week to four to six months depending on the seriousness and the client's response to it. Have they recovered their ability to walk, eat and care for themselves, for example? Have they stabilized? From a Shiatsu perspective, how robust is their Ki? Once qualified, and with time, especially with years of experience under your belt, you can start to sense when it is sensible to offer Shiatsu touch and the relevant degree of pressure or energetic penetration. To use or to give it, it is likely that you will have some considerable Shiatsu experience before you start working in this field, or that you will be under the guidance of a teacher or other mentor if you do not. It is hoped that you will be offered supervision or have made your own arrangements.

Move through your normal opening questions and diagnoses. Once you have the measure of the Ki state, you will know what can be done and what should be avoided. Please note that deep energetic work can be as exhausting and inappropriate as strong pressure if the receiver is frail and already managing high doses of post-operative medication. Approach slowly and keep grounded and centred, especially if you are working on a hospital bed and in an environment full of extraneous demands, and only penetrate deeply if you do so with an open awareness and in resonance with the client. If you feel distracted, ungrounded, very upset emotionally or if you are questioning what is happening, it is better not to give. Either take a break, perhaps walk around or practise some deep breathing, maybe speak with the client, staff or family about how the client is coping. Then reassess the situation.

Client awareness and feedback

Drug levels can be extremely high – both for physical pain and mental agitation – so your client may not be able to give you feedback or make decisions for herself. Some clients ask for a stronger touch if they have a neuropathy (lack of sensation in the area), but not always, and be careful as this can result in a worsening of the discomfort.

If you think that your client is unable to make judgements about their pain levels, whether or not it has been acknowledged by others, you must not treat. If, however, you are familiar with your client from previous sessions and you judge that they are able to give you adequate feedback, you can trust yourself to give Shiatsu. The usual rules apply: that you can only work with someone who can give you permission to touch them, or when someone else who has been empowered to make decisions for them has given you the go-ahead. It is likely that you will be in contact with family members and medical practitioners in a way that you would not be in your clinic and when working one to one, and they might be able to tell you how the client is and what medications they have had. They may give you permission on the client's behalf or ask you to do something to contribute to their care.

There are documented, difficult situations in which medical and other health professionals are asked or it is demanded of them by the relatives to do something which is close to being against their code of ethics, professional or personal. Examples of this would be to rehydrate in the very last hours when it is clear that this would actually cause the patient distress, and be a sort of reversal of the natural progression of death. For us as Shiatsu practitioners, it is unlikely that this type of thing would occur, but it can happen that the client has asked you as their trusted therapist, well in advance, to be with them at the end. The family, either not knowing or not understanding, might contradict this, not wanting a stranger there, wanting privacy, or being generally or specifically concerned. Therefore, you may want to consider making a written agreement in advance, when the client is of sound mind, and having it witnessed. You might also discuss whether a family member could be present, or part of such an agreement, when you sign it. Ultimately you are bound to your client unless she is no longer in charge of herself and a Power of Attorney has been granted to someone. In that case, you must comply with that person.

If you are working with someone who is at the end of her life and knows it, speak together about what she wants to happen if she loses mental awareness. Check whether Power of Attorney has been granted to someone, and what should happen in the eventuality of loss of consciousness or death during the Shiatsu session, for example who to contact in addition to the doctor. As for agreeing a will, you two can formulate a plan and write down the details of her wishes regarding you and her treatment up until she dies.

For confidentiality after death and issues regarding client records, please see Chapter 5, The Practitioner.

— Chapter 3 —

Life-Threatening and Terminal Illness, Loss, Grief, Shock, Pain and Trauma

Grief and loss are covered in this chapter, together with the responses to being given a serious diagnosis, trauma and shock.

Life-threatening and terminal illness

Many clients behave as if life will never end. If we were to confront them with how short it might be, they would admit that they know that, but the way they live often assumes that it will go on forever. People assert that one must assume that, as life cannot be lived in fear. It is often not until a client meets death, either personally or in their work, that this changes. Then, there can be a different sort of awareness and necessary adjustments might be made.

Sometimes coming close to death does not make a difference.

When I first met TL, a heavy smoker, she was making frequent trips to the hospice to see her father who was dying of lung cancer. She explained that her grandfather had died the same way the previous year, as had an uncle. She volunteered the information that they all took him outside in the wheelchair when they visited him with the grandchildren 'to join him for a fag'. Once I got to know her, I did ask if she was planning on stopping, but she shook her head, 'I sorta tried after ma granda', but I was too sad.' She declined Shiatsu.

And sometimes it does!

KT was diagnosed with a brain tumour and immediately had her driving licence taken away. She chose to come for Shiatsu on the day she received radiotherapy because she relied on friends to drive her into the city. She not only wrote and fulfilled her bucket list, going places she had always wanted to go, but she also visited each member of the family to make amends and heal wounds, and raised an enormous sum for a new brain scanner at the hospital where she was being treated. When she was close to the end of her life, three years later, she was told that the consultant she saw on her very first visit thought she would not live longer than three months.

Getting a terminal diagnosis will disturb life for most clients, and, in some cases, a change in behaviour can seem to create extra time.

Change

For all these clients, expectations have to change, at least in the short term. They will have less energy and so cannot expect as much of themselves. They may feel less emotionally resilient: not be able to be patient with the children or watch the news without crying, for example. There are other considerations: perhaps they have to cancel a holiday because of treatment and will therefore lose money or miss out on the fun. Life is interrupted, sometimes abruptly, and Shiatsu can provide some support during this transition. It can be grounding at a time of fearful change, while at the same time acknowledging the loss.

Being positive, being honest

There is a balance to be struck between positive and negative attitudes when facing serious illness. Supporting clients to find what is right for them can be hard. We all run the gamut of emotions, from feeling fed up, angry and negative about the future, to behaving in an upbeat way and getting on with life. There is evidence to suggest that a positive attitude aids healing, and so there are health workers of all types who promote this, even in the face of honest comments: 'I feel lousy,' said one client, as I walked into his room at the hospice. 'Never mind,' replied the nurse who was helping him get dressed, 'tomorrow is another day.' It can be a relief for our clients to talk about how they really feel, as long as they can be reassured that it will not hinder but help their progress. It can have the added benefit of helping their loved ones understand and know how to help them. Training ourselves to hear the bald truth takes practice and self-reflection, but it is very important if our clients are going to be able to tell us what they need to. It can be upsetting for all concerned, so each practitioner must make their own decision about how to manage this.

Sorting out the past

There is no doubt that many at this stage of life are concerned with how they have become so ill and are going over things which happened in the past. Even in the face of their serious condition, some have an impulse to look back at the past, to examine their and others' actions and search for understanding and forgiveness. In a state of health, when there is apparently time, this personal journey of discovery can unwind gradually. However, at the end of life, clients can feel the imperative for this to happen quickly.

YR was nearing the end of life and increasingly unable to go out or do the things he used to do. With extra time on his hands, his thoughts were turning more and more to the past, to what could have been, and he was angry. Very young, and pressurized by his mother to marry the mother of his soon-to-be-born, unexpected child (the result of a one-night stand), he gave up the love of his life and did as he was told. Sixty years later he needed to speak out loud about his unhappy marriage, and above all of a pregnancy termination which he had discovered his late wife regretted and about which he had never spoken. The words spilled out of him, repetitive and full of emotion as he received Shiatsu.

Control and independence

Almost everyone who faces serious illness has to ask for help more than they used to. The fiercely independent clients often feel helpless. Their previous image of themselves changes as they struggle, and this can engender a sense of loss. Slowly, the client must integrate this new, more dependent aspect, or at least there seems to be a connection between doing this and achieving a positive outcome such as a 'good death' or remission.

It is worth noting that the style of Shiatsu, where the client directs what happens and calibrates the touch and pressure at each stage, might be more useful for these types of people than another. The client has a rare opportunity to feel his own power and make his own decisions, changing his mind if he wants, with a practitioner who is open-minded and focused on supporting him to feel empowered. For a brief time, he can get a sense once again of his old self, perhaps even believe that this period will pass and he will get well.

Being in hospital or the hospice can be infuriating: people come in and check bloods in the middle of the night; the temperature in the hospital is higher than at home, so sleep may be a challenge; and the client cannot necessarily keep food down. Private parts of the body are touched by practical hands. When facing some of the things associated with having a terminal illness, it takes so much energy to hold on to being in charge and staying on top of things – even the strongest have to give in and let some things just happen around them. Understandably, this can raise more feelings of frustration, even anger, in our clients than it would do for those who are more laid back by nature. If we are invited to visit, we can follow the Ki instinctively. We can also use the Large Intestine meridian, we can encourage them to do breathing exercises and focus on the exhalation, we can listen to their feelings, work Small Intestine to help them sort out when to fight their corner and when not, and give Shiatsu which puts them in touch with their whole self to enable priorities to be established.

Embarrassment

Those clients who worry about what others think of them may suffer embarrassment if they have to ask to have their nose blown or if someone has to wipe their chin for them after eating. The added ignominy of certain side effects (losing hair, steroids causing an increase in appetite and consequently weight gain, for example) makes it even harder. The positive side is that families can draw closer, and the client discovers that people keep on loving and do not abandon him, which may have been an underlying fear prompting previous behaviour patterns. This can happily result in a valuable change in attitude.

If Shiatsu was part of a person's life before, then sessions will take them back to a familiar place and that could be reassuring; if not, then being treated gently and having their needs met on a deep level will help with managing these transitions.

Role reversal or change

Role reversal or change is usually hard to accept and upsetting. Shiatsu honours all the stages in the cycle of life, including middle and old age. To start as a dependent newborn, move into and through independence, and then become more dependent again, is simply part of life. However, it can also be hard to bear.

BB has bowel cancer and told me that the day before the session he soiled himself in his daughter's house. He was distraught. 'Having it happen at all was bad enough, but why did it have to be there?' he asked rhetorically. 'She already has the baby's nappies to change.' He did add that his daughter didn't seem to mind, which might have helped a bit (and I said a silent thank you to the daughter for that, as it must have been very hard for her). During the session, he was able to express some of the complicated feelings around this situation. The Spleen in the Hara and legs addressed the incontinence and helped him accept what was happening, and the Heart meridian supported him with his upset, hopefully aiding the integration of this and the wider situation, so that he could move on.

Afterwards

Although the client hopes that life will resume without change, in fact this is impossible. What is usually meant by 'getting back to normal' is that the client is hopeful that certain things will not change, for example that they will be able to go back to work, or start exercising again. Sometimes this does happen – the surgery and chemotherapy are successful and the client moves into remission; but at other times it can be 'wishful thinking' and they know inside that life is going to take a different turn, or that they will die soon.

Removal of body parts

Breasts, bones, blood and limbs can often be replaced, organs too in certain cases, but other aspects of physical normality – nerves and lymph glands, for example – cannot. In more than 90 per cent of cases, the client will choose medication and/or treatment and they all have side effects, some more debilitating than others. Having body parts removed will always involve loss and resulting grief, though clients will revive at different rates depending on their resilience and ability to accept what is happening, combined with awareness and support levels.

Clients with genetic issues

There is an increasing amount of research being done into genetic diseases. This now means that a woman related to a family member with breast cancer may be told what the likelihood is of getting it herself and may choose to have a single or double mastectomy, causing physical as well as mental and emotional loss.

There are other genes that are passed on from father to son. While it is useful for Shiatsu practitioners to know where we stand on this, enabling us to approach the situation with clear Ki, as with all ethical issues it is not our place to decide for our clients if that is a good thing or not. When they make the decision to have surgery (or if they decide not to), the client will be dealing with fear of death and, possibly, the loss of at least one female family member to the disease. The spouse, children who are old enough to understand this (and know that they have this ahead of them), and other relatives, particularly the older ones if they feel responsible in any way, will all need different sorts of support if they attend Shiatsu. Once again, this multiple death and loss situation requires tender care.

If the parents or caregivers are not speaking to their offspring about these types of situation but you know the children understand and are fearful, you will have to decide what to do. Supervision and talking to colleagues will help you make a decision that works for you.

Loss

Sean O'Hagen (2017) wrote in *The Guardian* about Kevin Toolis's book *My Father's Wake*. He used a phrase that expresses the enormity of loss: '…the tidal pull of capsizing grief are the moments that resonated most with me, not least because they bring home the state of utter incredulity – and unpreparedness – that a death unleashes in those close to the deceased.'

Loss is the state of not having something you once had. It happens throughout life – none of us escapes ageing, sadness or fear of death – and we all move through the stages and cycles of life. We say goodbye, we move on, we let go, easily or with difficulty, or somewhere in between.

Here, we start to name some of the situations in life when change occurs, bringing loss of what was, and perhaps grief, together with a need for mourning. Let us look at these in more detail.

Distinctive types of loss

Some believe that the first scream or cry which accompanies birth is the recognition of loss of the safe environment of the mother's womb. The mother is no longer pregnant and that might be a loss for her. If it is the first baby, the parent(s) are no longer two, but three or more instead, constituting a loss of couple-hood. The person attending, the birth partner, may suffer trauma if it was an emergency or the first time they had seen someone in a lot of pain, especially someone they love. In some instances, the birth may have gone differently from what was expected, even resulting in death of the mother or child.

Death of an infant

The next few paragraphs are about the death associated with childbirth and babies, and the reader may be forgiven for thinking that it is a common occurrence, which is not the case. While it is in no way meant to cause distress, it may be upsetting to read if you have been through such a situation yourself or are planning to become pregnant.

I was working with a group of new mothers and their babies. The group was arranged by one of my former pregnant clients and, although they did not all know each other, many were friends or had done prenatal classes together. We did not do much Shiatsu in the first class, as is usual, but focused on cementing the group, agreeing aims, going over oils and so on. What we did was the breathing preparation for the mothers, making first touch, and the Hara strokes. Between the first and second class, one of the babies died.

The grieving mother took the time to write to me later. She said she was carrying the baby in a sling when she became distressed. They rushed her to the hospital where she was put in a life support unit, but she did not survive. The mother told me that she had been able to do the breathing, make the first touch and then give some Hara Shiatsu through the sleeves in the sides of the life support unit and had therefore been touching her when she died. She wrote about how glad she was that she had attended the class. I continued to visit the family in their home afterwards to give Shiatsu to the parents and sibling.

For many parents and grandparents, the death of a baby or child is the worst type of death they can imagine. There are different sorts:

- Miscarriages usually happen around 12 weeks, but can be later and are usually more significant if the baby has to be birthed naturally.

- A stillbirth is when a baby is born dead after 24 completed weeks of pregnancy (National Health Service 2019).

- Infant mortality is when a child dies before their first birthday.

- Child mortality is when a child dies before their fifth birthday.

- Children (of any age) can die before their parents in an accident or illness.

The mother could be a wide range of ages, as could the father, and such events will affect many people around and in contact with them, including those who are not connected as friends or family. There are other aspects of pregnancy and birth which may involve loss: premature babies where the parents will be fearful; complications with the foetus or mother during pregnancy; a baby being a different sex from the one desired or expected, and so on. I refer you to *The Stress Matrix: Implications for Prenatal and Birth Therapy* (Castellino, Dr R. 2000).

With some Shiatsu practitioners now training to be birth doulas, or otherwise becoming confident with neonatal and postnatal care, there is the possibility that we may be asked to attend a birth and witness a death or near death situation. Being present at both the beginning (or expected start) and end of life, you will form a strong bond with your client whatever happens.

Termination of pregnancy

If a woman becomes unexpectedly pregnant and does not want to continue with it, she may or may not have a legal right to terminate that pregnancy depending on where she lives, her ability to travel to somewhere where it is possible and finance it, and her religious or ethical beliefs or those of the community in which she lives. The levels of loss and grief she feels will be individual and reliant on other things such as her age, support structure, the circumstances of the conception, who the father was, health, wealth, work, family and so on. If she has more than one during her reproductive life, her circumstances and responses will probably differ each time. It is important to note that despite making the choice, the woman may still grieve and feel loss for the baby ('I know I did the right thing, but I am sad'), and the anniversary of the termination date may be a date she remembers.

The woman who decides to continue with the pregnancy may grieve for the loss of her previous vision for her future ('now my studies will have to wait' or 'now I will be a single mum, which was not what I had planned'); and the father, if he knows about it, may have wanted something different from the mother, and be grieving himself. Much later in life, if for some reason the mother and father did not have children but would have liked to, then the memory of the situation may reappear and be especially poignant.

Working with loss of a baby or infant

I have found that if a parent wants to retell the story in which they or their child faced death, and embodies it as they do so when the baby or child is present and actively included, then it can be very powerful. This can be done either as they are receiving Shiatsu or in conversation using different techniques such as mirroring, modelling and Clean Language. The child has the chance to relive the incident, perhaps for the first time, and to respond. For example, a baby will often cry at the moment when the mother describes him getting stuck in the birth canal when the midwife panicked because his oxygen levels went down. He may be on her lap or lying next to her on the futon in the foetal position, and acting out with her in some way which we can then work with if necessary. We can apply pressure to his head (if it was an occipital presentation birth) to encourage him to find his way out of the fix and find a new way to move himself down and out of danger.

In this manner, birth can encompass death and if not acknowledged might cause problems later on for those concerned. It is worth finding ways to communicate how useful Shiatsu can be to deal with these issues. Although cranio-sacral therapy is often used, we have a wide range of tools available to us, such as working in the combined Ki field and timeline (a Quantum Shiatsu technique) simultaneously with whoever is present.

DM brought his four-year-old daughter to Shiatsu because she had chronic constipation, despite being treated with very high doses of laxatives at the hospital. We devised active games to play with her for relaxation and to stimulate her bowel, and things improved. However, the father believed that the breakthrough came after the session in which he told me about an incident in which he had had an epileptic fit. He and his wife were walking and he had the child on his back when it happened. His wife had helped, but it was the child who had been in physical contact with him when he staggered and fell against the fence. As he relayed the information to me in the session, the child stopped playing and listened intently. I included her, acknowledging her part in the incident. He explained that his wife had been very scared and had to attend, in the first instance, to him and not the child, to avoid more serious consequences. I used the client's own words in my responses to this story, but also mirrored his daughter's movements, calling attention to them as well. Once I had ascertained the meridian patterns the little one was exhibiting, I had a clue as to what I could teach him to help her: different games to address the Ki, and later he taught them to his wife. She did them daily with the girl with the result that the constipation improved and there was no need for medication.

Loss is part of life

There are countless stages of the life cycle which may involve loss: the cessation of breastfeeding, putting the child in their own bed if they have been sleeping with the parent(s), going to school, moving through puberty, work, relationships, menopause and old age. Most are inevitable if death does not interrupt earlier, and therefore we must acknowledge them.

MH heard that the two daughters of one of the mothers at her children's school had died in a car accident while with their aunt and uncle. The deceased children's parents were left childless, and while MH did not know the family well, she was truly shocked. Her own two daughters were of a similar age and she found that the incident was on her mind during the day, interrupted her sleep and became the subject of many conversations. She became very scared for herself and her family. Although she came for Shiatsu over 20 years afterwards, she said that she felt the same physical sensations as she had at the time. The fear and pain returned when she had grandchildren and she had never shared it with a professional care worker before. Now in her late 70s she had developed kyphosis, perhaps a sort of armouring behind her heart, there was considerable sinking in her epigastrium, and her shoulders were stooped – a classic posture associated with a Metal element deficiency.

Loss of goals or ambitions

A long and healthy life, trekking up Annapurna and having a productive retirement are the kind of goals and ambitions which, when unrealized, cause loss. Political and climate change can result in plans being scuppered and human rights being denied. Losing hope can result in depression and desperation, but Shiatsu brings our clients back to their body, puts them in touch with small things like having their feet touched, feeling the weight of a leg as you lift it. For a moment, they know the way the world is again and this moves them towards a recovery of hope. Hope is a positive thought for the future usually based on a reliable past, and this will remind clients that some things are the same as they used to be.

Grief

Thea Bailey (1999) wrote about grief: 'And then there is the time of grief and shock, which leads to exhaustion, and we become vulnerable to emotions and a sense of emptiness. We struggle and don't know how to release our anger and tears.'

This section describes grief, its stages, the way grief is related to the manner of death, whether the body is present, and the effects on the client – what Shakespeare called, through Hamlet, 'the suits of woe' (Alexander 1951, p.1031). There is reference to some of the different types of people whom our clients will mourn and how their response relates to who they are.

There are other references to grief throughout the book, notably in the Five Element (Metal, Water and Wood) sections of Chapter 2; and please refer to Chapter 5 for a section on the grieving practitioner.

Grief is a response which a client has to someone dying and is usually marked by sadness. It is a complicated part of living, it changes us, and we do not recover from it in the way we recover from influenza. It covers a wide range of responses. It can be short or longer term, disappear and be triggered later, postponed until 'a better time', or maybe not expressed at all. Your client may be disbelieving or in shock, the realization dawning in small, perhaps manageable, chunks. There may be nightmares in which the client is trying to save the dying person from death and failing. It can result in terrible loneliness. Even when time is going by and the people around have forgotten what happened, the client's suffering can still be debilitating. We practitioners will not know the progression until it unfolds, but it is useful to know some of the possible variations and theory behind them.

Grief and TCM

In *The Foundations of Chinese Medicine*, Maciocia (1989, p.139) writes that 'the Corporeal Soul is directly affected by emotions of sadness and grief, which constrain its feelings and obstruct its movement', and because of the connection between the Breath and the Corporeal Soul, it stands to reason that those emotions have an effect on the Lung function too. Though effectively describing what we recognize as a deficient Metal element, this affects all the parts and therefore the whole. We must remember that grief and sadness are also present in everyday life. They are a way of stopping the other emotions getting out of control and are therefore normal and necessary. Grief and sadness are said to regulate and stop the overflowing of extreme joy.

TCM offers exact instruction for *right grieving*, and, indeed, any more sadness than that is wrong, so the texts state. It is good to hear that grieving takes time, a long time by our modern accounts, and that after that, one may need support. Some US doctors are currently prescribing antidepressants a mere 30 days after the death has taken place.

Five Element stages of grief

Nicola Pooley (2000, p.12) writes eloquently about the power granted to the Metal element – to yawn – and how it relates to grief: 'If we can yawn, we can be fully present in our breath and in our life. This enables us to acknowledge our own mortality. This is highlighted when we are bereaved. This grieving can include grieving for our own mortal state, as well as grieving for our loved ones.'

You may find that your client is passing through different stages of grief associated with the Five Elements (see Table 3.1).

Table 3.1: Five stages of grief

	Stages of grief	Element
1	Initially being at home with the rest of the family, coping with the practicalities in a grounded way. She takes care of others.	Earth
2	When they leave she is alone, privately grieving. Perhaps she struggles with no guidelines or rules to follow to manage her feelings. When friends call to see how she is and she tells them how lost she is, she feels their withdrawal because they do not know how to be with, or what to say to, her. She stops communicating. Depression may manifest.	Metal
3	She reports a sort of death in life or confesses that she is willing her own end, asking, 'What is the point?' She says that if death is so close, then she might as well just go for it and die herself, perhaps her time has come and she should re-join the universal stream of pure energy.	Water
4	As time goes by, she starts to take risks, lurching forward from high to high, perhaps to avoid the reality, maybe over-drinking, taking drugs and embracing hedonism. Alternatively, or following this, there may be a period of becoming re-acquainted with herself, as if from the beginning again. Using creative ways to deal with what she has been through, she might find she starts to feel glad to be alive.	Wood
5	Finally, she realizes that she has learned a great lesson from what has happened and feels wiser as a result. Transformation has taken place and the experience is integrated.	Fire

Note that grief may follow the Creative/Shen cycle of the Five Element phases, but if there are extremes it is more likely that the Control/Ko cycle will feature. An extreme withdrawal may affect the Metal element to such an extent that it causes the Wood element to go out of balance – into substance abuse, for example – jumping the Water stage. Clients can also move back and forth between the elements, or the phases may overlap.

Zen Shiatsu and grief

Working with clients using Zen Shiatsu usually involves working from a back or Hara diagnosis, even if the practitioner knows that grief is the primary symptom and that there are meridian functions which theoretically pertain to certain aspects of grief. You will see from Table 3.2 that all the meridians can be connected in one way or another, so in the absence of a diagnosis these can be used as a starting point. Begin by locating the symptoms in the table and working those related meridians. That will give you time to settle into yourself and then you can follow the Ki where it takes you.

Table 3.2: Grief in Zen Shiatsu

Lung	Separation from the deceased. Grief over not seeing the person again and not doing the things you used to do with them. Association with the father.
Large Intestine	Crying, screaming, wailing. Talking to others about the one who has died and how you are. Withdrawal and lack of communication. Depression. Alienation, 'No one else understands.' Feeling alone, 'I am not her son any more, I am an orphan.'
Stomach	Supporting others. Cooking for them. Being grateful for others leaving food for you. Needing hugs and family, especially mother. Coping with the practicalities. Relief – I am independent again, relieved of caring duties.
Spleen	The taking in of what is needed to survive. Supporting or not caring for the self. Going to ground, staying at home. Overeating to fill a space, or unable to eat. Feeling the lack of the deceased's support and care. Inability to care for others such as your children.
Heart	Happier memories starting to replace the ones associated with the illness (if there was one) and death. Recognition that the deceased is no longer suffering. Understanding what has happened to them or where they have gone. Religious or spiritual awakening, or loss. Integrating it all and becoming a new person as a result. The Shen becomes scattered: unable to sleep or feel calm.

Small Intestine	Mentally sorting things out: for example, thinking, 'She was old and was suffering, so now it's a good thing she has been relieved of that.' Dealing with their belongings: what to throw away, give to others or charity; and what to keep as mementoes. Making sense of the emotions.
Bladder	Fleeing from the awfulness of what happened with fantasy, suicidal thoughts or actions. Nightmares. Fear of being alone, of being unsupported. Shaking and shivering.
Kidney	Fear of what might happen if the self and other loved ones die too. Lack of impetus to eat, work, see others, take care of self. Wanting to die. Inability to move forwards.
Heart Governor	New and appropriate methods of protection – a balance of time alone and with others. Support from outside and in. Managing without the person being there for you.
Triple Heater	Hypersensitivity to those who have trouble knowing how to behave with you, for example when they mention the deceased or do not mention him, and when they ask whether you are okay now, or not referring to your loss at all. Immune system issues.
Gallbladder	Anger that he has died and left you alone. Frustration with bureaucracy. Fury over hospital or others' treatment of the deceased or of you. Doggedly suing for compensation. Making decisions (or not being able to) about any changes which have become necessary, such as giving the deceased's clothes to the charity shop or making a new will.
Liver	Inability to plan or make plans for the future. Making a new start with a burst of great energy. Resorting to substance or alcohol abuse. Swings from lethargy to activity, from one mood to another, from reacting in a confrontational manner to saying nothing and venturing no personal information and holding back.

Expressions of the Zen Meridian pairs

You can also use the expressions of the meridians with grief. Nicola Pooley (2001, p.21) writes:

> So, in practice, after diagnosis I have a silent conversation with the client's Ki. If the Large Intestine is Kyo, I imagine the client yawning and I sense for a level where their Ki starts to harmonize. It may be… working on issues of death and life. The movement which leads to a sense of most harmony is the place where I try to work.

Yawning is the expression of the Metal element.

Examples of Kyo-Jitsu interactions for different aspects of grieving

If the grieving client appears to be coping with everyday life but seems depressed underneath, the Hara diagnosis may be: Lung Kyo, Heart Jitsu. If the client is lethargic and unable to go to work or do daily tasks, but seems off-hand and could be masking significant isolation: Large Intestine Kyo, Bladder Jitsu. If the client says, 'No one would care or notice, so what's the point?': Kidney Kyo, Spleen Jitsu. For 'I wanted the voices in my head to go away': Large Intestine Jitsu, Heart Kyo might be the Hara diagnosis; and finally, if what the client declares is 'The kids will be better off without me ruining their lives', then perhaps you will find Bladder Kyo, Spleen Jitsu. Please note that getting such diagnoses does not mean that that client is suicidal, nor does it mean that if you do not get one of these that the client cannot be suicidal. This issue is complex and variable, and, as always, each client must be treated as an individual.

Feelings associated with grief

Your client may have feelings which are recognized as a feature of grief:

- Confusion – immediately after the death.

- Disbelief and denial – 'I can't believe it, it can't have happened.' The grief can shield from the enormity of the loss in some ways.

- Unreality – a sense that it was reversible in some way.

- Numbness – related to the early stages of shock, perhaps. 'I feel nothing, I am unaffected by life going on around me, I do not smile when I see that the sun is shining.' This is often found alongside denial.

- Escape and avoidance – sometimes this offers some respite (and is different from denial as the mourner knows that the death has happened, but is choosing to engage in activities which allow them to get away from it).

- Obsession – thinking about the loved one all the time (and their possessions) is a recognized response. This is also a form of avoidance.

- Trying to be strong – sometimes this protects for a while, but it is not appropriate to stay in this state in the long term.

- Guilt – a sense of 'What if I had done something different?' or not done, said or not said. This is related to bargaining, one of the key stages.

- It's not fair, with more questioning – 'Why? He was so young, he had so much ahead of him.' This is also related to bargaining.

- Anxiety – the body's natural response to danger or a threatening situation.

- Loneliness – a feeling of being horribly alone and without the loved one.

- Shock – can be characterized by numbness, a lack of emotion and sensation. Also, by shallow breathing or holding the breath, an inability to communicate effectively or take in what is happening elsewhere, stillness or shaking or periods of both. There is a sense of being both incredulous and unprepared.

- Trauma – the effects of severe emotional shock and pain.

- Desperation – 'I want to die (too), to be with him, to avoid this terrible suffering, because that's all I can do.'

- Fearlessness – 'I have nothing to lose except life. I might as well live it to the full and do what I always wanted to do.'

- Wondering – when they will start to have memories from 'the old days' and not just the final period if it was distressing, they may think that nothing will ever change and be right again.

- Relief – 'Thank goodness he is at peace', 'I am so happy not to be caring for him any more', 'I am so glad it was not me.'

- Learning – 'Death is just part of life.'

- Resignation and acceptance.

Behaviour associated with grief

The client's behaviour can be varied. They might:

- be compulsive

- not be able to let go of the deceased person's belongings

- have memories going around and around

- be 'seeing' them, talking to them, looking at their photo and touching their things, visiting the grave

- not be getting out of bed/off the sofa/out of the house

- not be eating, or change their diet and eat a lot of sugar and takeaway food, resulting in illness

- not be feeding other people, animals or plants who or which are reliant on them

- not be keeping themselves or their surroundings clean and tidy

- be unable to work and lose track of the time

- change the way they do things to try and make the parent proud of them and, conversely, have a sense that what they do does not matter because the parent is not there to acknowledge it

- become aware of mistakes which were made and wish that they had done things differently

- feel extremely alone and emotional, as if the world is falling apart around them, and cry a lot

- feel that others who are alive seem distant and uncomforting

- feel that others are not appreciative – that if their parents (or children, friend and so on) are still alive, they need to be reminded that they might die soon and that they should appreciate them

- feel as if a gap has opened up, have a sense that something vital is absent and even that they are becoming a different person.

Jamie Anderson (2014) writes of grief:

Grief, I've learned, is really just love. It's all the love you want to give but cannot. All of that unspent love gathers in the corners of your eyes, the lump in your throat, and in the hollow part of your chest. Grief is just love with no place to go.[1]

It is worth noting that crying and feeling as if it will never stop, feeling alone, missing the person who has died and a lack of interest in life are all a normal part of an appropriate response to someone dying. Clinical depression (CD) shares many of grief's symptoms, but the latter may come and go, for example being manageable when at work, but feeling unbearable in the early hours of the morning or on an anniversary, whereas CD is unchanging or worsening.

Physical symptoms associated with grief

- Constipation, skin rashes and other signs of not letting go.

- Back and neck pain, urine infection and other signs of fear.

- Cramps and other signs of anger.

- Headaches and digestive issues and other signs of over-thinking.

- Shoulder pain, locked jaw, shallow breathing and other signs of shock.

- Herpes and fungal infections such as thrush and other signs of not looking after themselves.

In the same way that we can explain a symptom like the common cold or a skin rash as being the body's way of trying to rid itself of both physical and other things which need clearing out, so we know that grieving is there for a reason, it has a function. Contrary to the above, clients may focus on the deceased, realize the extent of their feelings, and take extra care of themselves and others who are alive as a result.

Spiritual responses associated with grief

- Loss, gain or change of religion or other spiritual beliefs.

- A sense that God has deserted them. Sometimes this faith returns and other times not, or not until just before the client's own death.

---

1   https://lessonslearnedinlife.com

- New understanding of what happens after death, perhaps as a result of being with the dying person, or as a way of making sense of what happened. This could be positive or negative.

- Loss of direction in life or reason for living. This could be temporary or even result in suicide or other type of death.

Layers of grief

There are layers of grief. The immediate stages can each take different amounts of time to pass. The life stages – birthdays, anniversaries, children's graduations or weddings and other family occasions – can be poignant. Death anniversaries are usually emotional events. For some, these events may be a joyous occasion, the family or friends having had time to come to terms with the death and accept what happened, so that they can celebrate and remember their loved one fondly; and for others it could be that even the second and subsequent occasions are worse than the actual death day itself – they may feel more alone. Making a record of the date in your client records, so that you know when it is coming, will aid understanding as the time approaches. If you find the client showing more serious signs of grief again, you will understand why.

There is grief which is associated with growing up and maturity – a parent's death may feel different to a young client and change as he gets older, for example, or feelings may be triggered by a subsequent death. Grief very often lingers for much longer than expected, and it is not at all unusual to start to work with a client who it transpires is still actively grieving someone many years later.

DC presented with chest pains. As the muscles relaxed around the upper back and thorax, he started to cry, something he said he never did, and then he spoke of memories of his long-dead father who used to take him on walks in the Welsh hills.

A client may start grieving before the person concerned actually dies. Their parent or grandparent who develops Alzheimer's disease, for example, may slowly stop recognizing them and become increasingly dependent. Thus, they might speak about gradually losing that person before they die. They may also be grieving the loss of the person who was in the caregiver role and acknowledge a swap from the child role to a caregiver or to taking full responsibility for them.

Different degrees of grief

It is sometimes implied that grief over the death of certain people is worse than others. ('Worse' usually means it is more violent and lasts longer.) The implication is that a cat is mourned for a shorter time than a child, or a client cries less for a friend than a grandparent, and objects are always bottom of the list. In practice, this is not the case and must not be assumed. It is the degree of attachment by the client which is important: a client may be much more upset when his dog, his faithful daily companion, dies than for a relative who lives many miles away and has not visited for many years. Sometimes, in fact, the client is surprised by the nature and strength of his grieving and only realizes how important that person/animal/thing was for him as a result of it. The house or item of jewellery which somebody is upset about losing usually points to an underlying situation, perhaps someone associated with the thing or item who is being mourned – someone has stopped visiting and the brooch is all they feel they have left, for example. There is also unexpected sadness for those with whom we have no easily identifiable connection, and yet we feel it strongly. The national mourning over Princess Diana in the UK is one example, as is the grieving for a favourite pop star, or the friend of a friend. Grief is complicated, and listening to the Ki is always the first job of the practitioner.

Withdrawal

There are many reasons why clients may withdraw, and it does not mean that they are not grieving. Some need to grieve with non-family members such as the Shiatsu practitioner, because there is a degree of objectivity and less of a worry that they will cause upset. Indeed, for some, the Shiatsu session is the only time they talk about it or that it is explicitly or implicitly shared. Their lives are busy or they are alone at home and perhaps it does not feel safe without someone to 'hold' them when they cry. Alternatively, being solitary can be the best place for others – the car parked away from busy roads for a short time, a walk in nature, even a swim in the municipal baths with noise all around, but no personal connections.

Keening, the sound of grief

Sikh women may wail, but are discouraged. It is the same for Muslim mourners, for it is the spiritual effect and outcome which is paramount. In the UK, displays of emotion are not encouraged either. Crying and keening are, however, natural responses to heartbreak, and Shiatsu can often free up the emotional expression.

My eldest daughter (aged five at the time) was close to her grandfather and wanted to be at the funeral. Family members were very unsure about this, but in the end the little one (six months) stayed at home with someone she didn't know – everyone she knew was with us – and my daughter held hands with her grandmother. In the silent church, she howled. It was the most terrible and appropriate noise and I will never forget it. I stood behind them and did not know if I should move forwards and take her out, but she just stood there until it passed. That was her own reaction and perhaps also she was expressing my mother's feelings too as the latter was her usual stoical self, holding it all together as she had been taught to do as a child during the war.

Coming back to life after grief

Sometimes grief can become a habit, and Shiatsu, because it raises clients' awareness of how they are, can help them recognize that they are in the recovery phase. When we work with clients who are grieving, we will be watching them find life again. Not everyone goes through the same stages of grief, but coming back from the loss of a loved one is usually gradual and continual. We hope it ends with the loss having been integrated and the client finding a new way to go on without them, although it rarely feels possible in the earlier stages.

Death of a parent

A parent dying is of course a serious matter and your client will react strongly one way or another, even if there has not been much contact for a while or there was animosity between them. If they were close, then finding a way back to some sort of normality may take much longer than they expect. Your patience and a regular appointment will support them when it feels as if it will never end and things will not be the same (which of course in one way they will not). If you sense that another session would be supportive, try to make a repeat appointment at the end of the previous one so that it is in the diary and they do not have to make contact to ask for help each time.

Shiatsu for grief

Shiatsu practitioners will identify and be able to categorize the signs of grief – sighing, sunken chest, downcast eyes, lack of vitality, facial pallor – according to theoretical knowledge. In grief, the breath becomes compressed, the Ki movement arrested, compacted and acting as a type of protective armouring. Grief affects the whole body, but is often located in the head in an unconscious attempt to reconnect with the deceased, and this can result in the closing of the lower energetic centres (with thanks to Blanche Mulholland). We will then have a range of possible touch responses and treatment plans available to us (see above).

Like a Gestalt cycle, a client can get stuck at one stage, struggling to move through it, and this may be when they seek our support. Stuck Ki will need releasing, perhaps to encourage the client to relax into gravity: in supine with the client's arm at 45 degrees from the side of the body, palm upwards, place one palm at the front of the shoulder (centre of the hand over Large Intestine 15) and the other on their palm. The Hara is positioned mid-way between the practitioner's two hands, facing the client's naval. Inhale and, then, lean forwards on the exhalation. As the bodyweight comes forwards, the practitioner's two hands move naturally away from each other and the client's arm becomes stretched in between. Repeat with two more breaths and on the other arm. While crossing over behind the head, alternate palms or thumbs can be applied to the Lung 1 Tsubos.

Exhausted Ki which feels as if it is worn thin will need to be met: using the edges of both hands, connect with the skin through the client's clothes. Delicately, working up from the pubic bone (Kidney 11) to the clavicle (Kidney 27), angle the pressure slightly inwards and down, as if the hands would join around four centimetres below the top surface of the abdomen and underneath the sternum in the thorax. Change the speed of the engagement to match the client's breathing rhythm, even if uneven. Repeat as necessary.

Grief is the natural response to a wide range of life events; it is complicated and unique, it affects clients differently, on all levels, and with various results, and it simply cannot be over-emphasized how beneficial it can be to offer your client space to express themselves or be quiet, whatever is needed. I have found that grief alters depending on who is hearing it – the quality of an attentive therapist's listening can be transformative.

Shock

There are many first-hand accounts from those who have had near death experiences and they often correlate with each other: life episodes flash in front of people's eyes, and there can be sudden realizations or revelations. The speed brings the potential for shock, but it is my belief that the one who is dying does not miss out on the stages that a slower death involves, it just happens faster. They see death coming, and the phrase 'time standing still', which many describe, is the organism's ability to manage everlasting time in the blink of an eye (like night dreaming) – now being explained by quantum physics. The person is conscious as it takes place, and consequently knows what is happening. I would venture, therefore, that a spirit does not get left behind or in an in-between place due to the speed of death. This is how it seems to me. For a selection of books on the subject of near death experiences, see the Further Reading and Resources section.

Shock is the first reaction to an accident, whether it is the person involved or someone who hears about it at some considerable remove. Unexpected and unwanted, these situations can result in the familiar grief and loss responses listed above, and the Ki is always in danger of becoming stuck like that if the initial state is not acknowledged and expressed. The Small Intestine is the shock absorber of the body. Carola Beresford-Cooke (2011, pp.231–232) describes it as an 'example of the body-mind's refusal to assimilate unacceptable information' and goes on to write about the possibility of symptoms remaining for years after an accident (whiplash is a common example). She adds that 'the Heart protector absorbs the effects of shock in order to protect the Heart'.

The situation in which the body of a client's dead friend or relative is not found may be the result of a natural disaster or war. There may be questions about whether they are really dead – sometimes it helps the client to see the corpse or to know that the coffin in the church or crematorium chapel has a body in it in order to integrate the reality of the death. If the ritual associated with the client's religion usually involves a wake, then the absence of the body is vital. For grieving children who did not attend the hospice or morgue, but last saw their parent/sibling at home alive, this can be a problem, even many years later.

Shiatsu, in these circumstances, will focus on what the client believes has happened, even if others give a different version of events. During the session, the practitioner can encourage the client to sense where or how the deceased person is and if that person needs to find peace. This is a process whereby the client connects with their deep knowing. If they can do this, you can work with that. If not, they will have to find a way to integrate the not-knowing into the bodymind, and perhaps the Heart meridian will be useful so that the client can carry on with life.

When I was working at the high security prison HMP Dumfries, giving seated sessions as part of a health event, the men confided in me. Their outer surface was hard when I touched and I had to use elbows as well as thumbs. Just underneath this tough exterior was an immense vulnerability, a sense I had of a great yawning space. I had an image of their Ki searching for security and comfort. I felt this with many of them. They were highly emotional individuals who felt that they were in danger when they returned home on parole. They appeared to have very few opportunities for this sort of support and I was sorry that the planned project did not go ahead so that I could return.

Tradition changes according to religion or culture. For example, it is traditional for Islamic mourners to bury their deceased within 24 hours where possible, except in the case of a person killed in battle or when foul play is suspected. In those cases, the circumstances must first be ascertained, but in the meantime, mourning is established.

Shiatsu and trauma

Shiatsu practitioners, caring by nature, are sometimes drawn to offer Shiatsu voluntarily. Richard Whiting worked at Refugee Advocacy, Information and Support in Lancaster, a drop-in centre for refugees and asylum seekers. He says:

> Clients were often suffering severe trauma, loss of home, and hardship. They had bodies of wood from their hard work and efforts to survive. We did not speak each other's languages, so the people could neither explain their problem in any depth, nor understand what I was trying to tell them. In the end, I just let go and put my hands on. (Whiting 2019)

Empathetic people will pick up stress and even trauma from a newspaper report, or can have a specific response to media coverage about a violent or particularly distressing death, so we and our clients may need support with this.

There are articles written about Shiatsu and trauma, and I refer you to those by Cliff Andrews (2018), Suzanne Yates (2018), Alice Gardoni (2018) and Peter Itin (2009).

Shiatsu in humanitarian or international aid scenarios

Shiatsu practitioners work in a range of humanitarian aid situations where death is a regular occurrence and loss a feature of every client case. On Lesvos, Greece, where Shiatsu practitioner Liz Sheldon works, many refugees are often stranded. Traumatized by the unspeakable horror they have witnessed, the journey, and grieving the loss of their land and home, most have post-traumatic stress or full-blown post-traumatic stress disorder, often with complex features. Only able to respond to acute medical problems, Liz has to practise Trauma Tapping (described as 'sensitizing acupoints and parts of meridians – in the face, hands, upper chest and sides of the body') rather than Shiatsu (Sheldon 2019). There are also practitioners and students working with Mission Shiatsu Humanitaire, a national government organization set up by the Brussels School of Therapeutic Shiatsu, which works around the world, notably in Senegal, with nurses, doctors and patients of all ages.[2]

Liz Arundel (2019) gave Shiatsu in Bosnia in 2000. She writes:

---

2   www.shiatsu-ebst.be

It was my first visit to a recently war-ravaged country and it was truly shocking. Most of the people we treated were 40-plus years old and they had the usual aches and pains like arthritis, but it was treating the trauma that was most needed, and their grief. We were there for two weeks so I only saw clients once.

Diego Sanchez (2001) was at Ground Zero after the 11 September 2001 World Trade Center attacks:

Immediately attending to urgent needs blocked much thinking out of my head and I just followed the flow and my instinct to help with touch. The firefighters who stopped by us immediately understood the benefit even the briefest session could have on their wellbeing and their stamina, and they would later come back with a colleague in tow… it was quite exceptional to see massage in an emergency life-and-death situation.

Pain

The sort of physical pain which the practitioner will come across when working with those facing death may be associated with cancer, angina (chest ache or squeezing sensation), and the burning or stabbing one-sided sensations which occur after a stroke. Ask the client to explain exactly how they are – do not guess or make it up, as there are safety issues and other contraindications to take into account. If the client does not know or cannot tell you, you can refer to a family member or health professional for that information, but remember that information coming from them will be coloured by their own perspective and approach. Even if you have a great deal of experience and knowledge, there are often new situations arising and new medical procedures being devised, so you cannot be expected to know it all.

Pain is fickle: sometimes it responds to touch, sometimes it abhors it. Focusing on pain by touching, or by thinking or talking about it, can help it to dissipate, or alternatively it can be exacerbated. Sometimes it is a good thing for it to worsen in the short term (with the client's permission, that is, if it is the result of something you did because they said it felt useful to them), but it may not be. Certainly, if there is a wound, there is no question of traditional Shiatsu thumbing on the site, although an exceptionally gentle palm may be positive. In such situations, working off the body could be more appropriate. In some cases, such as back pain due to a weakening of the bones from cancer, osteoporosis or medication, it could feel beneficial to the client at the time, but cause worsening in the days following. This may mean that the client refuses further treatment in the future.

Dealing with pain can bring clients into their physical self, or it can have the opposite effect where they retreat into thoughts to get away from it. In general, pain's function is to call attention to something which needs to change, so the practitioner's job is to find ways to accompany the client back into her body. Your concentration on the painful area allows for different options: it lets the client recognize the shape and size of it and describe it, which might mean that they make adjustments as a result; it takes the client's awareness there so that she can direct you accurately; and it allows her to make connections between that place and other areas of the body, thoughts and emotions.

It is very hard to focus on anything else when one is managing extreme pain, whether acute or chronic, and it is usually exhausting, with a good deal of mental worry attached to it. Remember to follow your intuition and never go against an instinctive sense that you should stop or change. Do not be persuaded to do something which does not feel wise.

Where to touch and use of the Mother hand

Take note of the Hara or back diagnostic area where you can or cannot touch. Being able to make contact with the Spleen area but not the Large Intestine, noticing that the Liver meridian is all hidden, but the Triple Heater is available, and so on – this is all very useful information about the client's Ki. Working with physical pain (maybe a scar, internal growth or swelling) requires a strong (but not necessarily heavy) and present Mother hand. This will convey reassurance and ground and centre both you and them. It may not be possible to place it on the Hara if there is a colostomy, ileostomy or urostomy bag, so it may be a matter of taking your time to find the right place elsewhere.

Temporal scanning

Temporal scanning is the work of Cliff Andrews (2004, p.11), and in this case he writes about pain in the joints: 'This is useful if I want to explore how the joint problem has developed over time. I can "feel out" the history, and in the case of trauma I have the option of treating back at the time of the accident.' This technique is applicable to other time-based symptoms or states of mind. It is surprisingly straightforward and quick, something which can be useful when the time allotted for a session in a hospice is very short, and a client is unable to tell the practitioner, or does not know, when was the origin of the pain.

There is a great deal more to be written about pain in the Shiatsu context, but these are some of the aspects which are connected with situations where loss or death are concerned.

— Chapter 4 —

The Client

Our clients are the focus of this chapter of the book. It looks at what they die of (the statistics part); where they die (including the definition of palliative and end-of-life care, plus all you need to know about attending a death); who they are (ages, stages of life); and how they die (by natural causes, either slowly or suddenly, and violently). There are some clients who deserve a special mention (people with disabilities, carers and medics); and a short section on how tragedy coverage in the media affects us all. There are sections on mental health, suicide and assisted suicide. Finally, we will address the diverse religions and cultural traditions in our shared community, and the use of ritual and rite.

Causes of death

Using 2017 statistics (the National Records of Scotland, the Office for National Statistics (England and Wales), the Australian Bureau of Statistics and the National Center for Health Statistics (US)), the biggest official causes of death in the English-speaking world are ischaemic heart disease (men) and Alzheimer's and other dementia-related diseases (women). Cancer (particularly lung and breast) continues to kill 28 per cent of the UK population, and one in two Australian men and women will be diagnosed with it by the age of 85. In addition, unintentional injuries, chronic lower respiratory diseases, stroke, diabetes, influenza and pneumonia, kidney disease and suicide feature in the list of causes of death.

While the infant death rate (that is, of those under one year old) is still much lower now than in the past (in the UK there were 6313 deaths in 1986 and 2578 in 2015), it has recently increased slightly in England

and Wales (2651 in 2016). Cancer is the most common cause of death for children aged 1–15 years, accounting for 20.6 per cent of deaths in 2016 (Cancer Research UK 2019) and 26 per cent in the US (National Cancer Institute 2018).

Where we meet those who are facing death or grieving

Death happens in many places and can take place at any time – most of us do not know when. The type and place of death has implications for the work we do with the grieving and bereaved afterwards. There are as many types of death as there are people in the world, and, like birth, none of us know how ours will unfurl. Even if we have warning or, rarely, have the privilege of planning our own, we will never know exactly how it will go. For those with an illness or disease, it could be that the family and friends do everything they can for their loved one, supporting them at home. Alternatively, a hospital or hospice is necessary or chosen (sometimes by the carers – medical or personal – and sometimes by the dying person themselves). Deaths which happen suddenly or away from home are very different from those which are expected – the practicalities and emotional reactions are different for those left behind.

Private venue

The most common place we see clients is in the Shiatsu clinic or private room, often in the practitioner's own home. Some new clients will come for the first time requesting support with a death or loss issue, and others will have been with you for a while when something of this sort occurs. We have the right to refer rather than treat ourselves if we find we are too upset (see 'Referrals, working with others and saying no' in Chapter 5).

Private clinic

Renting a room in a multi-disciplinary clinic or a specialist Shiatsu centre creates a different situation for clients who are facing loss. These premises may have more of a professional atmosphere, with a reception area for waiting and support staff to offer a drink of water afterwards, call a taxi or proffer a paper hanky.

Clients facing death and loss may be emotionally precarious, requiring stability and consistency from the practitioner. To avoid having to find a new room at short notice, a contract with the clinic owner is absolutely essential to protect you and your clients, however awkward it feels to insist on one. Running your own clinic gives increased freedom, but brings its own practical concerns.

Client's home

In someone's home you can move the furniture to obtain access to give Shiatsu, and will possibly have less time pressure, depending on your client load and other commitments. At the end of life, in the client's personal surroundings, it is likely that the Shiatsu will support your client to take their own time to die in their own way, if that is the stage they are at.

Health centres, spas

In the UK, health centres or spas are places where those who are not at work come for relaxation, to fortify themselves or regain health. That may include clients who are facing death and loss. Health spas in the US sometimes offer Shiatsu, as well as Watsu (Aquatic Bodywork)[1] and Five Element massage, acting more like a health clinic.

Independent

In the UK, there is a current growth of independent businesses, especially not-for-profit and community-based, which seek to offer affordable Shiatsu to those on low incomes. As 'The mortality rate from avoidable causes is more than three times higher in some of the most deprived parts of the country [UK] than the most affluent' (Holder 2018), we are more likely to meet death while carrying out this work.

Corporate work

It is less likely that those who know they are dying will be found in corporate settings. However, many of the people you work with in such

---

1   Worldwide Aquatic Bodywork and Therapy: www.watsu.com

venues will be managing grief or illness, fear of death, or ongoing loss associated with life changes. With medical developments in disease management, there is a growth in the number of employees who are receiving treatment for cancer and chronic diseases while remaining at work. There have been attempts to bring a spirit of preventative health into the office or manufacturing environment.

The open air

Many clients want Shiatsu when they are at festivals, markets and in other open-air or tented scenarios. A question about alcohol consumption, a contraindication, will have to be on the short questionnaire they fill in before the session, even if it is a seated session. There are often children who are keen to receive Shiatsu in these types of places.

Setting up my stool on the Meadows in Edinburgh, a large open space, one spring, I noticed a gaggle of young boys watching me. After smiles had been exchanged, one approached to ask what I was doing. He listened intently and consulted his siblings, before asking if he could 'have a shot'. I explained that there should be a parent or other adult present and he explained that they were all working on the fair rides across the green, but he ran off to ask permission and someone briefly came back with him to agree. As we were in the open air for all to see, and the other little ones were watching avidly, I decided it would be okay to go ahead even though the adult had returned to her work. The boy loved it! His wiry, taut frame was most responsive; he closed his eyes and really entered into the experience, while the others told me about their travelling life and how they go to school during the winter, when they settle for a few months. Throughout the day, different members of the clan came along to kneel and 'be done', all on the recommendation of the first young lad. I pieced together a collective tragedy from scraps of information about an uncle/brother/father who had died in an accident. I had the sense that between them they were carrying the loss, sharing it and managing together to keep the good memories alive. It was one of my first experiences of giving Shiatsu to a group who were so closely linked that there was a sense that touching one of them had an effect on the others, and of how closely the Ki is shared in such life and death situations. I know now that it is not unusual for the young ones to be the catalysts for the larger group to get external support.

Hospital

There are three reasons for a practitioner or Shiatsu student to be in a hospital setting if they are interested in working with those who are facing death: volunteering or working; at the invitation of the client or client's family member; and treating staff, relatives and carers. Around the world there are reports of individual projects where the practice and research of Shiatsu is being carried out in departments ranging from intensive care to cardiac departments, in oncology, paediatrics and pain management. We work with patients who are dying, scared they might die during procedures, or suffering unexpected complications after treatment.

Due to insufficient official evidence that Shiatsu is effective and safe, it is not routinely offered to patients or prescribed as part of primary care. However, the public (including off-duty medical staff and their families) use complementary and alternative medicine and are generally positive, increasingly providing 'anecdotal' evidence, requesting information from doctors and taking up the voluntary therapies on offer – they 'vote with their feet'. A few private insurance companies (in the UK) are consequently reflecting this by allowing people to claim for complementary and alternative medicine (Health Shield and Elect, at the time of writing).

In Austria, students from the International Academy for Hara Shiatsu (formerly known as the Hara Shiatsu College) have been working in hospitals for some time. Tomas Nelissen (2005, p.3) wrote: 'With the clinical practice we want to prepare the students for their practical work. Our interest in the hospitals lies in the opportunity to deepen and strengthen our capabilities by working with clients with clearly defined patterns.' Their work is 'with the human being as a whole. …there is no aim to treat diseases or symptoms. From thousands of treatments we have learned that there is also a remarkable improvement in the symptoms of the clients.'

Allopathic medicine divides the body into systems; there are separate medical clinics and units dealing with them. This approach may be less likely to attract Shiatsu practitioners who work with the whole bodymind unless they are already qualified medical personnel. Janice Fennell trained in both gastroenterology and Shiatsu and works as a clinical nurse specialist with inflammatory bowel disease (IBD) in Scotland. She shares an example of Shiatsu for pain management:

> I was asked by nursing management a few years ago to do Shiatsu on an IBD patient who specifically requested complementary therapy. I needed to show management my Shiatsu qualification and insurance. I have known the young patient for many years so we had already built up a trusting relationship. Shiatsu was the only thing that influenced his pain. He had been on strong opiate medications for his IBD for many years. Giving Shiatsu on a hospital bed was certainly different, but a good experience. I had to keep the sessions to no more than 20 minutes' duration as he was acutely ill. I think it was important that I was doing the sessions in my IBD nurse time. (Fennell 2019)

Some Shiatsu practitioners work in recovery: after radio- and chemotherapy; once a cardiac or renal patient has been stabilized; in rehabilitation; and with chronic rather than acute presentations. In these situations, almost everyone will have faced death in one way or another, sometimes thinking it is imminent when the hospital staff know that it is not, as this is not always clear to the patient. Due to the high levels of anxiety and the stressful environment, our results are almost always positive: it is the way we touch, our lack of intimate intrusion, our ability to make deep contact quickly and our flexibility to be able to work with what is presented that make us welcome. Expectations are often low: the medical staff do not usually think we will make a difference to the trajectory of the pathology, and thus we can be left alone by them to get on with the job of calming and listening, which we are so good at. This is not to under-emphasize what we can offer.

There are major differences for the Shiatsu practitioner who works in these situations:

- The emphasis is on disease and illness, rather than health and wellness.

- There is a focus on curing, rather than self-healing.

- The medical procedures take priority over Shiatsu.

- The medical staff do not necessarily know or trust Shiatsu.

- The environment is not conducive to a calming of the nervous system.

Now, let us look at our relationship to this sector from another angle. Government services are looking for new ways to meet patient demand and demonstrate financial discipline. Examining the most recent National Health Service (UK) reports, we can see that they are written in language which we recognize. The Scottish Health and Social Care Delivery Plan (Healthcare Quality and Improvement Directorate 2016) states on page 2, 'By 2021...more people will have the opportunity to develop their own personalised care and support plan.' In section 10 (also on page 2) it goes on, 'To improve the health of Scotland, we need a fundamental move away from a "fix and treat" approach to our health and care to one based on anticipation, prevention and self-management.' In point 24 of that page it states that it aims, 'to expand the multi-disciplinary community care team with extended roles for a range of professionals...to develop and roll out new models of care that are person- and relationship-centred and not focused on conditions alone'. And finally, underneath point 24, the Scottish Government states, 'We will achieve this by...supporting development of new models of care.' We have pioneered this approach, which will help patients if implemented. If we want to work in primary care, it is necessary to understand the requirements of the health services and find ways to share our knowledge. If we are able to demonstrate that we can fulfil these aims, there is more chance of integration.

Hospice (government and charity)

Holistic medicine is better understood in hospices. Patients are treated differently: the emphasis is on shared care with teams of health professionals which often include complementary therapists (CTs). The focus of CTs is on symptom control and relief, principally of cancer, but also of other terminal or chronic illnesses such as lung disease (chronic obstructive pulmonary disease and emphysema), multiple sclerosis and Parkinson's disease.

Shiatsu is relatively unknown and it takes time for it to become accepted by both the CT and the primary care teams. Obtaining work in a hospice will usually be via written application and interview, and we must, therefore, rely on our credentials before having the chance to demonstrate with touch. We must find ways of proving with words that Shiatsu is safe and effective, that we are well trained and informed, and are prepared to work alongside others in a complementary rather than alternative capacity. In my experience, making claims for which we cannot provide evidence and using terms such as 'healing' are ineffective.

Later, giving bodywork sessions can be very useful, so our colleagues can feel what Shiatsu is and, themselves, recognize the effects. As we settle in and the work progresses, the staff begin to receive feedback from patients and to understand what we do. We are then more able to use the skills we have. Being flexible and humble is important, as it is we who are being accepted on their terms.

One impressive aspect of primary care settings is record-taking. Bowel movements, drug levels, mood and behaviour are regularly noted in detail. This means that we have unusual access to data showing the results of our work – the short-, mid- and long-term results. Over time and with growing confidence, we have the option to point out the sequence of events: how often the constipated client has a bowel movement after a Shiatsu, is calmer, or sleeps better, waking less often to call for drugs.

Sometimes, however, the opposite happens: there is an acute or disruptive episode following a Shiatsu session. Because of our status, staff will not usually identify a connection – their focus is on medication regimes, the progress of the disease itself, and other interventions. We know that our work causes change, and indeed sometimes the patient can articulate this. However, consummate skill is necessary to explain this to hospital staff without causing alarm.

TX presented with lung cancer and asked if the Shiatsu could help with his back pain. When I saw him the next week, he told me that he had been admitted to hospital the day after the session where they tested him and discovered that his lung tumour had increased and was pressing on his spine. This resulted in him receiving different and more appropriate treatment. He wanted to tell me that it was the Shiatsu which had alerted him, before the hospital had done the tests. He was convinced that it had been useful, but if the medical staff had made the connection between his treatment and the hospital visit, I might have had some explaining to do.

We have various options. We can use the data and patient feedback privately within our own community until we are confident that we have a fully comprehensive explanation (that symptoms sometimes worsen, prompting a new diagnosis, resulting in increased support for the patient) and until we have enough to provide the impetus for further research; or alternatively, we can continue with our work and see what transpires.

It is vital that we keep accurate and appropriate client notes for the primary care team so that they know what we do, and in case of prosecution. Establishing methods to record patient feedback and results is vital if we are to identify suitable areas for, and contribute to, research in the future. It is advisable that feedback from the patient's family and friends is also included.

In the hospice, clients may be cared for by other specialist caregivers and it is useful for us to understand their roles:

- Nurses from Marie Curie (a UK charity) assess and carry out care planning. They are qualified and registered. Marie Curie healthcare assistants are trained to follow a code of conduct, and give care in the client's own home, especially overnight in the case of those with a terminal illness (not just cancer) (Marie Curie n.d.).

- Nursed from Macmillan (a UK charity) work in hospitals as well as in the community. They are specialists in cancer and/ or palliative care, with skill in pain and symptom management, psychological care, assessing complex needs, and advising other health care professionals (Macmillan Cancer Support 2017).

- Community district nurses (UK) assess, monitor and provide health care. They are employed by the NHS and have a palliative care remit (Duquesne School of Nursing n.d.).

- Community nurses (US) are caregivers, educators, monitors, advisers and leaders across the areas of health including mental health. They work with the community in places such as prisons. They are employed by the state health departments (Nursing Times n.d.).

When in the hospice, it is most useful to be part of a complementary therapy team, where you will have some shared understanding of theory and practice, although with differences according to modality; or in a mutually accountable, multi-disciplinary patient team made up of you and the staff of the medical institution where you are working. You will be able to access notes and information from other team members, including doctors, nursing staff, consultants, physiotherapists, community nurses, occupational therapists, psychiatrists, counsellors, art and music specialists and the chaplaincy. Working as part of such a group is usually a positive experience, although it takes time and diplomacy to communicate and learn how to work in this way.

Joined-up care means there will be an element of mutual education between staff: we, the Shiatsu practitioners, expand our knowledge of medical procedures and current practice; the primary care teams learn about holistic Shiatsu and how we value and promote health.

Charity-run organizations

Shiatsu is routinely offered to clients, their families and carers in speciality, charity-run, premises for those who are HIV positive, or have Parkinson's, multiple sclerosis or cancer (see the Maggie's Centres[2] and other cancer care centres). Much of this work is voluntary.

Other

There is a history of Shiatsu in head injury units, homeless hostels and clinics, alcohol and drug dependency units, young people's centres and day centres, often provided by students on final-year placements under supervision. Those dealing with accidents will have faced death, and those involved in addictive activities that considerably hasten death also fall under the remit for this book. Practitioners working in places where young people are involved in gangs know that there will be a lot of fear about knife crime.

End-of-life, palliative care and attending a death

In the US, there is a distinction between palliative care and hospice care. When treatment ends and there is nothing more that the doctors can do to keep the patient alive, palliative care begins, but treatment

---

2   www.maggiescentres.org

can be carried out in both circumstances. In the UK, palliative care is part of end-of-life care. Technically, palliative means to relieve pain. It includes treating symptoms and side effects, but not addressing the cause. Palliative care aims for the patient to have the death he wants, to remain conscious and pain-free, and to be able to live fully until he dies.

The goal of palliative care is to achieve the best quality of life for patients and their families, and to provide a support system to help patients live as actively as possible until death (World Health Organization 2002). Although symptom control may be the main focus, there is also an emphasis in palliative care on patient dignity, autonomy and self-efficacy (Lu, Doherty-Gilman and Rosenthal 2010).

The definition of 'end of life' ranges from the final years of someone's life, to their last months, days and hours. The aim is to ask the client what he wants and to support his friends and family too. The hope is that he can live as well as possible until he dies with dignity.

Experiencing a *good death* at the end of life is the optimal goal of palliative care. Studies show that the meaning and description of good death varies across cultures in different populations.

Wishes at the end of life that defined a good death for the participants in the *What Matters Most at the End-of-Life for Chinese Americans?* study by Lee, Hinderer and Alexander (2018) (of 60 Chinese Americans in Maryland, US) included being pain-free, not being a burden to family, being with family, having a trusted physician, maintaining dignity, and prayer.

The Scottish Executive (NHS Education for Scotland 2006, p.4) has stated that 'spiritual care, which includes but is not limited to religious care, must be provided in an equal and fair way to those of all faith communities or none' and has developed culturally appropriate standards as a result. The Scottish hospices have adopted these, and the chaplains who work in them are familiar with the various specific cultural needs and respectful practices.

Please refer to Table 4.1 which summarizes the distinctions between hospital treatment, end-of-life, palliative and hospice care. It applies to the UK and the US unless otherwise specified. Sources: the National Health Service (NHS) Lothian, Scotland (2019), and the National Institute on Aging for the US (2017).

Table 4.1: Detailing distinction between treatment, end-of-life, palliative and hospice care (for the UK and US unless otherwise specified)

Medical treatment is:	End-of-life care is:	Palliative care is:	Hospice care is:
Given to patients with cancer, multiple sclerosis, Parkinson's and more.	Suitable for all types of patients.	Suitable for all types of patients.	Suitable for all types of patients.
For the patient.	For the patient and their families.	For the patient and their families.	For the patient, family and friends.
Curative, that is, treating the cause.	A curative treatment to relieve the pain and treat the symptoms and side effects of medication.	Providing pain relief and symptom treatment for medication side effects.	Providing pain relief and symptom treatment for medication side effects.
Offered at a nursing home; hospice for a short visit to assess the level of support and medications needed; hospital; or at home.	Offered at a nursing home; hospice for short visit; hospital; or at home.	Offered at a nursing home; hospice for short visit; hospital; or at home.	Offered at a nursing home; hospice for short visit; hospital; or at home.
Started as early as possible to identify and diagnose illness.	Usually only offered for a few years, months, days, hours.	Started as early as possible to identify and diagnose illness.	Offered only after curative treatment ends.
Provided by health professionals (including Macmillan (UK only)), community (district) nurses.	Provided by health and social care professionals, including community nurse (treatment and prevention).	Provided by health and social care professionals (Macmillan (UK) who care for cancer patients only, and Marie Curie (UK) for care for all terminal illnesses), friends and family members.	Provided by visiting health staff (Macmillan (UK) who care for cancer patients only, and Marie Curie (UK) for care for all terminal illnesses), friends and family members.

Offering chemotherapy, radiotherapy, other medication, other therapies such as physiotherapy.	Offering chemotherapy, radiotherapy, other medication, other therapies such as physiotherapy and complementary therapies, counselling, chaplaincy.	Offering a team approach to chemotherapy, radiotherapy, other medication, other therapies such as physiotherapy and complementary therapies, counselling, chaplaincy.	Offering other medication, other therapies such as physiotherapy and complementary therapies, counselling, chaplaincy, song, art, occupational therapy. And is 'holistic – physical, psychosocial' (US) and 'integrating the spiritual' (UK).
For short stays in hospital or hospice – usually not long term.	For short stays in hospital or hospice – usually not long term.	For the short term before discharging back to community.	For the short term before discharging back to community or 'before death' (UK); and 'within six months of death' (US).
To allow people to live with a life-threatening (US) or life-limiting illness (UK).	To allow people to live with a life-threatening (US) or life-limiting illness (UK).	To allow people to live with a life-threatening (US) or life-limiting illness (UK).	To allow people to live with a life-threatening (US) or life-limiting illness (UK).
To make careful assessment.	To respond to the wishes of the patient and family.	To relieve and prevent suffering.	To relieve and prevent suffering.
To help patients understand their choices for medical treatment (US).	To help people live as well as possible until they die with dignity.	To help people focus on quality and affirmation of life.	To help people regard death as a normal process.
To provide hope for a cure (US).	To provide care whether or not the patient is expected to die soon.	To neither hasten nor postpone death, but to give care whether or not the patient is expected to die soon.	To give care, although there is acceptance that the patient will die soon.

The UK and Australian health systems now publicly state that they offer treatment and support *whatever the cause*, and this could actually be seen as a breakthrough in the relationship between mainstream medical thinking and Shiatsu. We and the mainstream medical staff diagnose in our own individual ways and pay attention to different factors, but we both recognize and respond to client need. We all accept that blame is not important, and that all people are equally worthy.

How does our work and attitude change when we are in a hospice?

Cat Westwood (2019), a practitioner from Norwich, says:

> In comparison to my normal practice, I have to be even more mindful about the small things at the hospice. For example, the way in which I would finish the conversation. I found myself saying, 'See you next time' and changed it to 'See you'. It sounds insignificant, but words and behaviour greatly impact on the whole treatment, if you are taking a holistic approach.
>
> The treatments I gave to patients at the hospice generally lasted 20–30 minutes as they got tired very quickly. Surprisingly, with all the support and care…the patients often felt a lack of touch from others, so Shiatsu was well received. They reported benefits with sleep, pain and getting comfortable. I also treated carers, family members and staff, which I found supported and held the whole community at the hospice.

Gabriella Agular (2015, p.10) also works in a hospice in the UK. She writes:

> I sometimes demonstrate some pressure points for symptom relief as it makes me feel that I am there with a 'tangible' purpose. I explain to the nurse I will try Large Intestine 4 for the constipation issue brought to my attention… When I get a chance to speak to the nurse the following week, she is happy to say it worked!

Where do our clients die?

Studies have shown that 80 per cent of Americans would like to die at home where they are less likely to receive unwanted treatments, and in the UK the figures are similar. However, there is a growing tension between these stated needs and the feelings of families who are often unsure if they can cope.

As Shiatsu practitioners, we will also be caring for the family and friends who might not feel the same as their relatives. A difficulty arises when the dying person wants to stay at home, indeed is told he has a right to do this, but the family are not keen. Perhaps his previous behaviour towards the rest of the family, his irascibility as a patient (on top of the practicalities of clearing up and looking after him), are more than they can manage in various ways. It is important to acknowledge this and be prepared to manage complex relationship issues as well as the physical, emotional, mental and spiritual aspects of the client himself.

Carers have to learn fast to manage the needs of someone with a life-threatening illness or at the end of life. In the same way that it is said that a parent must be doctor, teacher, counsellor, personal chef and chauffeur all rolled into one, so for an end-of-life carer the skills are multiple. To understand the funding system, the medications and need for house alterations; to undertake the nursing, cleaning, food provision and listening; to manage the daily cycles which are more like those of an infant than an adult – with night waking, possible incontinence and mood swings – is a significant litany of tasks for anyone, even a loving and willing client, never mind if they have children, a job, or are old and unwell themselves. To provide Shiatsu at home, maybe for both the principal carer and the dying person, would be ideal, but unless they can afford to pay you for your extra time and travel, or you subsidize it or find an alternative source of funding, those people will miss out if the patient dies at home. There may be a need to run basic Shiatsu courses for carers so that they have some extra resources to support themselves.

Wherever they are, the care team will have to negotiate their way around the needs of the dying patient and those of the family who would be his full-time carers. Some people in a hospice, hospital or residential facility do not want to be there. This is not because the 'system' does not facilitate it, nor because the family are too busy or uncaring, but because sometimes people take a long time to die and that may mean many more years of looking after someone who has not supported the family himself. We hear stories of people who have divorced or separated, but then find themselves looking after their 'spouse' before death. They need quite as much support as the dying person themselves and we must understand the complexity of their duty and emotional connection. If the patient gets what he wants, dominating the needs of the carer(s), the latter will have an extra layer of grieving when the time comes – for themselves *and* their lost time and energy.

Professional carers, the staff who work at the care homes and those who help people at home are generally very poorly paid. Furthermore, their workload is heavy, including early mornings and late nights, with changing schedules and transport problems. It does not give them or others a sense of their true value. Unskilled in medical matters, but highly skilled in the practicalities as well as the psychological ways of dealing with folk, they might be the only day-to-day contact for someone who is housebound. As well as the cleaning up they are employed to do, these staff might experience racism and themselves come from families who need help. Generally, they are neglected by the State, employed by private agencies and cannot afford Shiatsu, even though they need us. We, in turn, may struggle financially to care for them.

Refusing medical treatment

Some of our clients may choose to eschew medication and surgery, focusing instead on letting the body take its course, or using complementary therapy and lifestyle changes instead. Relevant books, articles and opinions abound. The internet is full of them and there will be plenty of opinions offered from the people who surround our clients on how to heal themselves from life-threatening illness. There will be some Shiatsu clients who ask us for advice. Some practitioners will be more comfortable with offering it than others.

The client may refuse medication and medical procedures if they have already undergone serious treatment, know what it is like and cannot face it again. Maybe they have been warned that their immune system is already impaired and therefore the prognosis is poor and the treatment would be a 'long shot' anyway. Perhaps they do not trust in what is offered; cannot afford it; do not have access to medical care; or this type of treatment is not compatible with their religion. It may be that they have a presentiment that there is no point. In most countries, including the US, a patient can refuse treatment that is recommended by a health professional, as long as they have been properly informed and are 'of sound mind' (Nordqvist 2018).

VR had breast surgery five years before I saw her for the first time. Her doctor was recommending that she had another operation, but the results had been so deleterious before that she had promised herself 'never again'. Now she was worrying over that decision. I did not see her for three months, and when I did, knowing that she had decided not to have the operation, I saw that she was close to death. She had lost a lot of weight and her arms were like birds' legs. Her eyes were sunken in their sockets as if they were looking inside. She said there was no joy. She looked keenly at me and asked me if I had joy in my life, and listened intently to my answer. She informed me that they had nearly lost her the previous weekend and we had a brief discussion about why she was still here – 'to see the grandchildren', she said. In between bouts of falling asleep, she refused Shiatsu, and said over and over that she did not want to stay 'on this planet'. As I sat with her a while, I became aware that much of her Ki was outside her physical body, about six inches (15 centimetres) away, especially around her throat and third eye chakras. We said goodbye and at the door I turned for a last look. She said, 'I will keep in touch', and I found myself blowing her a kiss.

In the UK, it is a criminal offence for parents not to seek medical care for their sick child. If they ask you for Shiatsu for the child instead of medical treatment, you should make sure that they sign a disclaimer, but you may still be complicit. You must tell them that it is your duty to prompt them to see a doctor.

Attending a death

A client who feels supported by you over a period of time, who trusts that you know him and whom you have helped manage pain and distress in the past may invite you to be there when he dies. It may be for pain relief or something else practical, or for mental, emotional and spiritual reasons. He may want to be as conscious as possible, to be close to the others around him, and to know what is happening when death comes. Maybe he is alone, or his family cannot or do not want to attend, or for some reason he does not want them to be there.

Carol Shuford (2019) writes:

I knew that working with those whose death was imminent would require facing each person with kindness, respect and a wish for their peaceful transition. I knew that at least during each session, I would need to be unafraid of death and dying and that my concern be placed on the preciousness of the life that still remained.

People can be nervous about touching or being close to someone who is dying. That is where the Shiatsu practitioner can help. If you have been invited then you can do the touching instead, but your job may be to support others in finding confidence to do it. There are simple pointers you can give: rubbing the hands together to warm them before making contact will take the visitor's mind off themselves and their worries; suggesting they ask permission to touch first, so they feel welcomed; and showing how starting by touching a hand, the hair or a shoulder, without any pressure to do therapeutic actions, can be very powerful. The client may be hypersensitive so that off-body or very light palming is best.

Shiatsu teachers often place hands on their students so that their experienced Ki can help the learner to connect and feel something. Shiatsu practitioners at the bedside can do this with others who are there. It can be calming for the giver to be touched by the practitioner, and at the same time be a way of encouraging someone who is inexperienced with touch to be brave and send their love through their hands. If contact is not possible, we can find ways to teach or show how to sit still, to be centred and present, radiating Heart energy into the shared Ki field in order to be consoling and complementary.

A client can be fully accepting of his impending death and want to spend some time with his friends and family to say goodbye, but be at a different stage of acceptance from them, which is causing difficulty and hurt. They might be struggling with the fact that he is dying, scared about seeing him (perhaps because he is thinner or scarred or otherwise changed), worried about whether they would say the right thing, or even that they might catch something and get ill themselves. Closeness to another's death inevitably connects us with our own.

The atmosphere at the bedside of a dying person can be light and frivolous, or emotionally tense, and it can also move between the two. There is a lot at stake. People may be overwhelmed, including the Shiatsu practitioner, especially if it is the first time in such a situation or there has been an upsetting experience before with someone else. If the person is being cared for by medical staff, they should not be in pain, but visitors might not know that. If the person is not comfortable, it can be highly distressing, upsetting and scary. Whatever happens, every moment will be precious and so it is almost always an intense and highly charged time.

The signs of death

It may be useful to know the signs of death so that you, the client and any others present can be reassured. One client said that her mother stopped moving altogether because her limbs were so weak. This is what happens: the physical body slows down, it is a mirror of what is happening inside as the organs cease to function. It is a natural, even a kind way of leaving – gradually – and, if possible, all present will recognize it as that and be progressively prepared. In the same way that we have nine months to get used to the idea that there will be a new member of the family during pregnancy, deaths of this sort come gradually.

Remember that you are an expert with Ki and it is very likely that you will intuitively know what is transpiring with this client, even more so if he is familiar to you. It is possible that the spirit leaves sooner than the body finally stops functioning, or that as aspects of the bodymind release, there may be a series of different Ki stages.

Medically, the systems start to slow down:

- The heart and therefore the circulation, although occasionally the heart rate rises.

- The pulse.

- The breathing.

- The bowels.

- The bladder.

- The kidneys, so there can be oedema.

- The muscles, so there can be difficulty swallowing (do not offer food or drink at the end unless the dying person asks for it, as it is the client's way of leaving).

- The nervous system, so being very hot is not uncommon.

- The lymphatic system, therefore the dying person will be susceptible to pneumonia.

- The five senses.

They may want to be alone, but also to see people to say goodbye. The client will sleep more. Please note that not all clients will have all of these symptoms.

The tongue may be black or darkish yellow and dry; the lips may turn outwards; and there may be a yellowing or flushed face (though not necessarily with a high temperature). There may be a paradoxical pulse.

There may be increased pain, but not all noises and movements are signs of pain. Instead they could be:

- involuntary, because the nervous system is deteriorating

- jerks, because the liver is struggling after a long period of high doses of medication. Note that this may be a sign to stop or reduce such medication

- memories which accompany emotions (and which might be described medically as delusions)

- visitations from 'others' coming to help them – it depends on what you believe

- an effort to communicate, which might become harder and therefore sound distressing.

Emotionally, there may be confusion, a readiness and welcoming of death, fear, anticipation and anger.

As the client relaxes, the domination of the disease recedes and the client can claim back their life. Strange though it may seem, this is a feature of the last moments. Eventually there may be loss of consciousness and then the last breaths, which may sound rattly if phlegm has gathered at the back of the throat and sinuses. You could sit the client up if that seems the right thing to do.

Any Shiatsu practitioner who has attended a birth or given a client some indication of what they are sure will happen in certain situations will know that things often do not go according to plan! Death is no different. Entering the room of a dying client, you may have an overwhelming sense of not knowing what to do, and that anything might happen before the inevitable. When you touch, that may change, and you might get a clear idea of what is needed; but it is common on such occasions for matters to take their own course. Our skill is to stay with them, chart what is happening in the moment, retain connection, acknowledge that it is beyond us, and be grounded.

How long will it take? That is unknown. Some have a miraculous recovery over a short or long term, others go quickly, and some die more or less at the expected time indicated by medical staff. What is commonly recorded is that in the same way a baby can 'wait' until the mother is ready, so the dying can hover on the brink of death if they sense that a beloved is holding them tightly, desperate for them to remain as long as possible. Thus, our work can also usefully be to support those around the dying person to take time to say goodbye, to hear any response, and then to let go. It can be very hard, and it is a skilled practitioner who can find a balance between the needs of the dying and of those by the bedside.

As the body enters the final stages, and the habitual, internal messages are dulling, touch and Ki can still be felt. It is wonderful to help someone release peacefully with a sense that you are present to 'hold their hand'. They will almost certainly know you are there.

Your emotional reaction to the death could vary greatly. If you are there in your capacity as a professional practitioner, you may manage to remain centred and be able to support those around the dead person until you leave. You may, however, feel moved yourself and this is natural. If you cry or find yourself expressing your own feelings, this will not be surprising and it may be appropriate – a human response. You may want to go away soon afterwards or you may recover and remain. Whatever happens, ensure that you give yourself time, and obtain support if needed, afterwards (see Chapter 5, The Practitioner). The results can be far-reaching, leaving you with a deep respect and also a sense of realism. It was a journey for you both and must be acknowledged as such.

Death doulas

Most of us are familiar with birth doulas – people who are trained to accompany women and their friends or family from the prenatal to the postnatal period. Death doulas are less well known, but are becoming more common. As a way of rediscovering the community role that a wise woman or man would have played in supporting the dying and their families in years gone by, an end-of-life doula seeks to aid a peaceful parting. A *death midwife* will help and encourage people to bathe, dress and mourn their loved ones at home if that is what they would like to do. It can be argued that fulfilling this traditional role is a natural part of bidding farewell and managing grief.

In the UK, the Crossfields Institute has established a non-medical diploma course of 20 days to inspire their clients to talk about and face death as a normal part of life. In the US, the Lifespan Doulas Association[3] created a training curriculum and is part of the National End of Life Alliance.[4] Death Doula Australia can support the client and family in finding new ways to approach death, provide a night vigil service (sitting with the person after they have died), and advice on green funerals (Love 2019). In an age when more people live alone than ever before, even in Japan where there is such tradition of families providing for their aged relatives, there are now what are called *lonely deaths* – people who die in their own homes and are not soon found. In response to this trend, Shiatsu practitioners who work with the elderly and death doulas have an important role to play in ensuring that their clients are remembered at the end of their lives.

The people we work with

We are all in the process of dying, and so you could argue that every Shiatsu session addresses this in some way. However, it is rarely spoken about unless there is a specific reason. We have examined what people die of and where, and this section categorizes our clients into groups for the purposes of examining the varying types of death, loss and grief we will meet in our professional lives. It looks at how we manage death among our friends and the fear that engenders, the loss involved in relationship breakdown and abuse, and how death affects babies and children. We also discuss clients who endanger their own lives or have dangerous hobbies.

There is a common belief that working with death is synonymous with end-of-life care, and that is certainly a major part of this book. However, as a result of my clinical experience and from listening to clients and other practitioners, I know that there are other situations and times of life when death also features. The aim is not to see death everywhere, but there are more people walking around thinking about death, or even willing it, than admit or say out loud. It would not be advisable to ask all your clients if they feel like this, but time spent thinking about some of these categories will be worthwhile, to prepare for the possibility of it arising in a session.

---

3   www.lifespandoulas.com
4   www.nedalliance.org

Clients with different faiths

When we work with clients who identify as members of a cultural or religious group within our community, it is respectful to research their traditions and practices.

The Sikh Missionary Society notes that care workers should be the same gender as the client, especially if the client or their family comes from the villages of the Punjab in Northern India. They caution us to be careful not to rely on the younger generation to translate for their parents and grandparents as it can be a real burden. Closely related to that respectful attitude is not making statements which assume something about the client, and not touching and behaving in a way which goes against their faith. In private practice, most of us attract clients who are from a similar background or culture. However, if we work with people who are managing loss in a women's refuge, hospice or hospital, we may meet clients from groups whose culture we have no previous experience of.

If we are not Muslim, there are important facts that we might not know: that Muslims prefer to give and receive things with the right hand, for example, and that most (not all) Muslim women will be happy to remove their hijab, chador, niqab or burka to receive Shiatsu from another woman as long as they are in private and no men can possibly enter unannounced. For this reason, it is useful to make clear on our websites and business cards that we are male or female as our gender is not always clear to everyone from name alone.

It is worth noting that Jews and Muslims forbid cremation, and either do not embalm or prefer not to. Knowing information like this avoids any disrespect when working with our clients.

These are just three examples. We are all advised to take care to understand clients who have religious or cultural backgrounds that are different from our own.

Clients with a disability

Shiatsu practitioners treat individuals, and Shiatsu itself is applicable to everyone. 'Disability' is a catch-all term dependent on different assumptions, historical terminology and culturally specific concepts. In searching for a way to distinguish between those who have and do not have a disability, I came across the phrase 'normal for a human being' from the International Classification of Impairments, Disabilities and

Handicaps (World Health Organization 1980, p.143). These words are used to make comparisons and therefore define difference, to enable fair treatment of all people and help them obtain the support they need. According to article 9 of the UK Equalities Act (2010) (United Nations. Department of Economic and Social Affairs, Disability n.d.) and the Americans with Disabilities Act of 1990, people with disabilities must be allowed equal access to services, so you cannot charge any extra for your travel time and costs if you are making a home visit. (You can decline the visit on the grounds of your own time and limited finances.)

In this book's context, there are specific death and loss issues which are relevant to clients who have a low life expectancy (for someone with cystic fibrosis in the US it is 37.5 years (Cystic Fibrosis Foundation 2017)); who require more frequent hospital treatment (someone with a congenital heart defect may require ongoing, life-giving or life-threatening surgery); or who need special protection in managing day-to-day activities and relationships (in 2016 it was reported that 'people with learning disabilities were 26 times more likely to have epilepsy, eight times more likely to have severe mental illness and five times more likely to have dementia. They were also three times more likely to suffer with hypothyroidism and almost twice as likely to suffer diabetes, heart failure, chronic kidney disease or stroke' (Learning Disability Today 2016)).

So, parents of children who are born with, or develop, a disability may often face death and thus seek Shiatsu for support. Focusing on one person in a session while simultaneously acknowledging the group field – parent, affected child, other siblings with and without disabilities themselves – is a way of managing such complex scenarios. You can either use non-touch diagnoses for someone who will not or cannot be still, or diagnose through the parent. Ask them to lie down, agree the aim, and then use your familiar touch diagnosis as if they are the one who you are treating. It is possible to give the whole Shiatsu by proxy too, if necessary.

Clients and birth

Expectant and new parents are sometimes fearful of infant fatality. Women from the poorest backgrounds and mothers from black, Asian and minority ethnic groups are at higher risk of their baby dying in the womb or soon after birth (Draper *et al.* 2018). Miscarriage, pregnancy testing, pregnancy termination and SIDS (sudden infant death syndrome, commonly known as cot death) all involve loss and death (National Health Service 2019).

Thankfully, in the Western world neonatal deaths are now rare. There is an infrastructure of medical help, patient support groups, charity guidance and back-up available. Thus, those offering pre- and postnatal care (an increasing sector in Shiatsu, thanks to the pioneering work of Suzanne Yates and Wellmother (Yates 1990)) will certainly fulfil a need.

Younger clients

Although the age difference between birth and 20 years is enormous in many ways, there are similarities in how babies, children and teenagers need to be treated when grieving. They will respond in similar basic ways to death in the family or to those close to them.

If a death is imminent, babies and children will be just as aware as the adults that something is wrong, albeit on a more energetic (pre-verbal) level. They will be acknowledging the coming change and grieving after whatever loss has already taken place. If it is their parent who is ill or dying, practical things will alert them: the parent may be in bed all the time, be worried, scared or angry, or be attending lots of hospital appointments; they may not be as able to care for the baby or child as before. There may be a more gradual shifting of childcare responsibility from that parent to others, but it will be very unsettling. If perhaps a sibling or pet is not there to play with the baby or child the way they used to, or is behaving differently due to disease or treatment, it will be noticed. The younger we are, the more reliant we are on smell, taste, sound and voice tone, appearance and body language. The changes will be apparent and, if unexplained or unacknowledged, will result in alterations in behaviour on the physical and emotional levels in the baby or child.

When the practitioner is attending the dying adult, the infant may be present. In this case, the Shiatsu practitioner can encourage him to tell his child what is happening and how he is. This is very often an unusual thing for him to do, but there is no doubt that babies and children are acutely aware of the energy of their caregiver(s), indeed they are totally reliant on it. If that person pretends one thing, but feels another, the young ones pick up this dichotomy. They become confused and distressed, showing it through eating, sleeping or behavioural difficulties. Babies are soothed and reassured by honest, congruent communication, and very often it is a relief for the parent too. As soon as the adult begins to speak, with our aid in amplifying the Ki in the room, they will usually witness the change in the baby. We can ask the adult to say how they think the child is responding and why, and we can point out the changes if they are not apparent to them, helping them make the connection between what has happened or been said, and those changes.

This also allows for explanation and reassurance. It does not matter if the child is pre-verbal. Babies are able to understand long before they can speak, and certainly before they can articulate complicated concepts in language. Anyone who has spent time with a newborn baby knows that they are alert to changes in atmosphere at the subtlest level. Thus, even if they do not understand the ideas, babies do know about mood. Having their special adult lovingly show or tell them who will care for them if or when they are not around to do it personally, that they will survive and thrive in the future, has tangible, visible effects on the baby. It is so very important for their survival beyond the loss, and we Shiatsu practitioners can play a large part in this, disturbing though it may be.

In addition, if the client can feel or name her own fear – of death, or of what will become of their child – in the Shiatsu session, it might of course be distressing, but it is real. Still very much connected to and relying on their sensations, babies recognize the Ki, in fact it could be said that *they speak Ki*. As the practitioner's touch connects with the client, as the client allows herself to release and feel what is happening, as the practitioner holds the space and allows the vibrations to penetrate the field in the room, the baby or child, the baby will know. Stopping what they are doing, they may crawl across to comfort the client, may cry, or alternatively fall asleep, knowing that they are no longer required to be vigilant and can rest because the caregiver is taking responsibility and being supported by the practitioner.

Therefore, the Shiatsu practitioner can do her work or ask direct questions in the child's hearing, and it will help rather than damage them. As the dying adult takes responsibility for what they are feeling, knows that it is their fear (that is, a negative projection into the future) and not a truth, the sound and energy of that will be understood by the baby, who can then relax.

All children can participate in the Shiatsu. In fact, it is helpful if they do. They like to give as well as receive, but they do not make a distinction between these two directions of Ki (efferent and afferent/ into and away) until they are older. Play is a broad concept, and giving and receiving Shiatsu comes into it. As the child interacts with the others in the room, they make intuitive choices, and acknowledge what their Ki needs for all to see.

Like pets, babies and children will direct the practitioner if she is open to this, and act as a sort of third hand – noting where the Ki is or is not and responding openly. When the practitioner allows for interaction, there is a wider chain of Ki exchange, and as the adult is usually the parent or primary caregiver, this will have been going on anyway at home, and is simply being made explicit through the Shiatsu, highlighting behaviour patterns and helping to identify causal factors. Thus, the emotional complications of death and loss can be brought into the Shiatsu room to be acknowledged, and perhaps also resolved in some ways – resulting, it is hoped, in the child feeling that he will always be loved whatever happens.

If the child is being brought up in a religious family, she will be familiar with the associated rituals from an early age and know what part she must play. Whatever transpires, the child can no more avoid the fact of death than the adults can, and shielding children from it can be damaging.

Given the chance, most children ask starkly direct questions about death when the time is right, suggesting it's good for them, and if allowed they will continue to do so. As they grow up and move around more in the world, coming into contact with those who have differing views and experiences, they will be able to formulate more complicated questions and comprehend increasingly in-depth philosophical answers. They will instinctively want to talk about and remember someone who was a feature of their lives and has died. If it is difficult to do this at home or with a parent or relative who cannot or does not want to hear, it may be during the Shiatsu session that this happens – whatever the age of the children or young person. This can make for a more complex session: the parent or another caregiver will be present, and so there will be a number of streams of Ki in the room to be managed effectively.

Children will usually not need to be reminded that life continues without that person or those people, but it may be important that the therapist signals that they should not be ashamed of that. Laughing, making jokes and playing at the same time as the dying process is unfolding and progressing is normal and their way of managing life. The Shiatsu practitioner, trained to be with a client in the moment and respect the state they are in then and there, can be a most valuable support at this time.

Some, maybe all, children or teenagers wish they were dead at one time or another, and that then their parents or carers would be sorry. These are real emotions and often a response to feeling badly treated or misunderstood. It is commonly a short phase, even if repeated. Although anything to do with death is important and should be treated as such when it is being felt, it is not the same as a suicide wish. They have probably not told anyone that they feel like this, and so may be isolated. You might experience this scenario through an adult saying they felt like this themselves in the past or that their child or one in their care has reported it to them. You may be working in a children's home or unit, or otherwise directly with the young person.

If there has been a suicide attempt or this feeling is related to an eating disorder, then the child will probably be under the care of a social worker, or you are likely to be working in a mental health institution where there is additional support and maybe medications are being administered. Children under the age of 16 rarely like to talk directly about such things. However, you are advised to say them out loud so that the children understand that it is possible and indeed healthy to talk about them. Shiatsu can be good in these scenarios because it can treat using games and pure touch instead of probing or pressurizing the client to speak. It is true that children are more sensitive to Shiatsu than adults, and they will respond more quickly and sense your care and support for them more readily. (There is a separate section on suicide below.)

If you are working independently, or in an institution where there is no record of the child being at risk, you must identify the situation you are facing: a morbid wish, a hard-done-by feeling (important, but not life threatening), or something more serious. If the child is under 16, there should be another adult in the room with you. If for any reason you are uncomfortable, seek professional support from Childline or a similar telephone support system run by people who are experienced in this area. You may even want to use the Emergency Services if danger seems imminent.

As mentioned, Shiatsu practitioners are in a prime position to support in this situation. If we have done our own soul-searching, we will know that human beings run the gamut of feelings and we will have considered our own childhood memories. If we have not, a client's case may trigger upsetting memories and these will need attention from you and maybe another.

Teenage clients

From 16 years upwards, young people can attend Shiatsu without an adult, and although most late teenagers do not want to speak about serious personal matters to their parents, they do listen, do need information, will have questions and may speak to a Shiatsu practitioner. It is most likely that an adult is paying for the session or has referred them, and you will probably therefore be briefed about the circumstances and reasons that Shiatsu was sought. Physical symptoms or insomnia will often be the limit of the information you will receive from them directly, perhaps a nod or shake of the head in answer to a direct question. It is best not to ask many. At a time when life is already all shook up and so many changes are taking place, loss and death are keenly felt and need to be integrated so that they can get on with their mission to grow up.

Witness the behaviour of teenagers after divorce: among all the loss and grief, what is still so important for them are their peer relationships, their friendships. If they trust that their primary caregiver is dealing with their own grief and situation, and if they are held tight, that is, looked after, given appropriate boundaries (not suddenly allowed to do anything they want, but kept within the routine and rules they are familiar with), and have the chance to communicate openly if they want to, then they can get on with making and breaking those friendships, keep on with their lives, and manage as best they can, when they are ready. Shiatsu is invaluable at this time, offering space and privacy, respect and support with practicalities that they might not otherwise get at home or in the place they live.

There are many adults who now choose to have counselling to deal with deaths they encountered as children. They would like some relief or to learn how to manage it better in their daily lives. There are counsellors who are specialists in grief for this reason, to support their clients through the results of new or old deaths. Shiatsu is not the same, but does something else – it acknowledges, raises awareness of the client's feelings, often situates them somewhere in the body, helps define the shape and density of them, and simultaneously integrates through the bodymind. In a Shiatsu session, the client is 'somatically experiencing their biological information', as Dr Cindy Engel wrote in the *Shiatsu Society (UK) Journal* (2018, p.6).

JG has a great many siblings and he told me that when he was at the bedside of his father, together with two of his sisters, there was a discussion about whether another who lived at a distance should be called. They agreed to do this, but the person chose not to attend. This caused difficulty for some of those present, but not for others, and as a result has been remembered. It was when I was giving Shiatsu to his left shoulder and upper chest during a time when his cough had come back that he spoke about it. At this time, their mother was nearing the end of her life and these memories resurfaced.

Adult clients

There are adults who do not or cannot face up to the fact of the death – a pet's, friend's or granny's – and maybe pretend to themselves that that person or animal has never existed. Perhaps they never refer to them and the message is clear – they ignore other people who do so. Then it can be the practitioner who diagnoses the gap in the Ki field and through his touch or the contact he promotes between those present seeks that which we all long for: some repair.

Clients whose parents die

If it is the last parent who dies, then the client will be an orphan and this is significant for some people, particularly if they do not have siblings or other family members with whom they are close. Not only has a beloved one died, but they are more alone, and perhaps the last representative of their family line.

Clients whose parent starts a new relationship

When a client's parent starts a new relationship after the death of the other, they may find that the loss of the deceased parent has been reawakened. In addition to the fear that they have now lost their living parent to another person, the family structure and allegiance will change, and anger and resentment may appear. There may be internal conflict between wanting the living parent to be happy, and a sense of loyalty to the deceased.

Parents who wish their children will die

Some parents wish that their children will die. They may live outside of the extended family for various reasons and have negative childhood experiences. It is extremely common for parents to feel overwhelmed and insecure. Usually these feelings are fleeting, but they are important and may be a sign of a severe lack of support, postnatal depression or other mental health issue. The parent will almost certainly feel ashamed of thinking these thoughts and try to hide them, or alternatively feel horrified by them and need to reveal them to someone.

Once again, Shiatsu practitioners are highly sensitive to undercurrents of feeling, and it is vital that we respect our own instincts, as this is where we are likely to pick up such information. This goes for all issues that clients are ashamed of or hiding. Transference is of particular note here: if you are giving Shiatsu to someone and find yourself feeling inadequate or bad, you are unable to get a diagnosis and do not know what to do to help them, and these things are unusual for you and your Ki is contracting (backwards and inwards) or you have a sense of disassociation or desperation, then something is probably wrong with your client which they are not telling you. You might need to gently break contact and go out of the room to assess and identify what is going on; to share what you are feeling or ask a question. Perhaps you silently take note and bring it up in supervision before you see that client again. Follow your Hara because it will reveal useful information.

Older clients

As we have seen, older clients may be in various venues. They will be aware of death approaching, if not their own then that of those around them. In Australia, life expectancy has risen to 85 years for women and 80 years for men, although this is lower for indigenous Australians by about ten years (Hospitals Contribution Fund of Australia 2019). The average is similar in the UK and the US; 18.2 per cent of the population is aged 65 years or over (Office for National Statistics 2018a), and dementia and Alzheimer's disease remain the leading cause of death for females in the UK in 2017 (Office for National Statistics 2018b).

Adapting your Shiatsu to work with this age group requires the usual sensitivity to the basic qualities of Ki. Blanche Mulholland (2012, p.10) writes: 'As an individual ages, the Yin energies increase at the expense of the Yang.' Bill Palmer (2011, p.6) agrees: 'As we get older the manifest (Yang) functions of the organism tend to degenerate. However...the quintessential (Yin) aspects of our energies do not need to dissipate. In fact, this is the time they can fully develop and supersede the physical functions.'

Clients who are medical students and staff

Shiatsu practitioners have often given sessions to medical students and staff in both private practice and in official institutions. Under enormous pressure due to long working hours and facing death every day, these people deserve our care. There are benefits to both of us: we learn a great deal about what they do, and they come to understand Shiatsu.

It is acknowledged that there is a fundamental lack of training for medical professionals in palliative care and in speaking with patients and relatives about their prognosis or death (Haelle 2018). Trainers are aware of this issue across the world and are starting to remedy this situation with postgraduate courses (some for up to three years, including placements).

Health workers are often prompted to start training because they want to help others. In reality, many find that managing what is required of them means cutting off from feelings in order to survive, and our theory and experience tell us that such behaviour can be injurious over time. This does not stop them acting with care, and we hope that the attention and understanding that we offer will begin to help them. In addition, perhaps there is a role for us to share how we protect ourselves and manage client work safely.

Look out for doctors and other health service workers who are not encouraged to show grief, but who do because they are human! Leeat Granek (2012) writes:

Our study took place from 2010 to 2011 in three Canadian hospitals.

We recruited and interviewed 20 oncologists who varied in age, sex and ethnicity and had a wide range of experience in the field – from a year and a half in practice in the case of oncology fellows to more than 30 years in the case of senior oncologists... Grief in the medical context is considered shameful and unprofessional. Even though participants wrestled with feelings of grief, they hid them from others because showing emotion was considered a sign of weakness. In fact, many remarked that our interview was the first time they had been asked these questions or spoken about these emotions at all.

Doctors have always been part of my client group and I have often been struck by the contrast between our training and theirs when it comes to emotional literacy and self-care.

Clients who are carers

Now recognized as a group with special needs, there are increasing numbers of carers of all ages in our population. The major charities recognize their requirements, hospices take them seriously, and young carers are identified in schools and colleges. Shiatsu has a lot to offer this group: a time and place to relax, someone to focus on and care for them, and an outlet for emotional expression.

Clients who have been abused

Abuse can happen in all types of relationships. People of all ages, races and social classes can be involved. Those who are abused may feel out of control, unsafe and angry. There are many aspects of abuse which are related to the topic of this book – the threat of death to the one who is being raped and others related to her, as well as feeling 'I might as well be dead' or 'I feel dead' after the event and even many years later. There is inevitable grief over the violation and loss of dignity and self-worth emanating from one asserting such power over another. While these feelings and type of damage are common to other death in life situations in some ways, there are added complications – potential or actual loss of money, job and affection, and maybe removal from the relationship. The possible resulting pregnancy, perhaps the loss of virginity and matters associated with that, birth and subsequent life all are matters which may involve grief, loss and death for the Shiatsu client.

Abuse is never justified. Listening to the Ki and/or using Clean Language and dialogue is vital to ensure that the client feels believed and respected. Care must be taken to ascertain the amount of pressure, to assess where, and indeed whether, to touch without re-traumatizing, and it should be recognized that even with permission this may happen.

In Portugal, 7 March 2019 was declared a day of mourning for victims of domestic violence after data showed attackers had murdered 11 women so far that year, the highest number in a decade (Almeida 2019).

The Reuters article which reported this went on: 'The charity, Refuge, estimates that two women are killed each week by a current or former partner in England and Wales – where the combined population is almost six times the size of Portugal's 10 million' (Almeida 2019). It is therefore not unlikely that you may see a client who is either facing such danger, or is a child of a woman who was killed this way. Such clients require the utmost care and you are well advised to involve other health professionals to support both you and them.

If the deceased parent abused the client, their feelings will be mixed and very hard to manage and they would be strongly recommended to also see a bereavement counsellor. As their Shiatsu practitioner, it will probably be helpful if you can readily accept the difficulty of loving and hating someone at the same time. This would be the same with a spouse or someone else who was expected to be safe and loving but was actually dangerous and manipulative.

Clients who struggle with accepting someone's death

If your client was away when a death happened and missed being at the bedside or the funeral, there may be aspects of denial, disbelief or guilt. One client told me about his father, 'I know he did die because my mother told me, but I am not sure I really believed it inside for a long time.' Similarly, after attending a funeral, the grown-up child of the deceased who moved away from home many years beforehand may find themselves grieving for longer than those who were present throughout the illness and at the time of death.

SA lived a long way from her family and there were no other close family members nearby. She said, 'The gaps between seeing my

dad were long before he died, so that every time I went back I
expected he would be there and he wasn't. I kept catching myself
thinking that I would phone and tell him about that thing I had
just seen that he would like...then I remembered he was dead.
The grieving seemed to go on for so long, longer than it did for
my sister who lived nearer and had seen him more often before
he died.' SA had no one close by to grieve with, and had to take
into account her small children who were coming to terms with
the loss of their grandfather, as well as her husband, who was
sad too. Shiatsu can support all concerned and it can be a good
idea to work with the parent separately, as well as together with
the child.

Clients whose relationships break down

Our clients move in and out of relationships all the time, as do we,
and the break-up of relationships with significant people – family,
lovers, friends – will involve a period of mourning. The length of the
relationship is not as important as the quality of the attachment, and
many things are tied up in the loss: the client's own health on all levels;
the effect that the relationship ending may have on the other people in
the client's life and their relationship with them; the future, including
issues such as having children or not; loss of trust; unpleasant social
and other media behaviour; and more. Some clients have resilience
and recover quickly, integrating the new information and reshaping
their lives; others will struggle to function normally for a long time.
It is important that the client as well as the practitioner respects this
timescale or the suffering will increase.

Relationship breakdown after the death of a child

It is, sadly, a feature of extreme grief, particularly following the death
of a child, that relationships fall apart afterwards. Like an explosion
going off in the midst of something, the family members can feel as if
they have ricocheted out in different directions and that there is no way
of getting back together again. Being with clients in these situations is
sensitive work and care must be taken not to offer advice.

Clients whose spouse or partner dies

The client whose spouse or partner has died while they had been living in the same house, with or without children, will have an added set of poignant situations to manage. Not only will there be grief, but everything around them will bring the deceased to mind. Initially this may be a good thing, but it may also inhibit a release when the time is right. If they were not married or their relationship was secret or unacknowledged (and this situation is familiar in the lesbian, gay, bisexual, transgender and queer or questioning (LGBTQ) community), then mourning with others, having adequate finances and having a place to live (if the house or rental agreement was in the other's name) may all be serious issues which will have to be worked through as time passes. Being sensitive and aware of the range of possibilities and associated feelings is of great import.

Clients endangering their own life through drugs, alcohol and smoking

People who do things that they are told will make dying more likely, or hasten death, are often keen to have Shiatsu. There are complex reasons for smoking, taking recreational or illegal amounts of prescribed drugs, sniffing glue or other solvents, and often drinking large quantities of alcohol. Many people find these substances are addictive, and almost everyone who behaves like this knows that they carry a health warning. Despite knowing this, there are a few who do it on purpose. They are very different from the clients who follow a predictable routine with minimal activity. We are trained to be highly observant, and we have strategies that make us sensitive to hidden signs. We do not ignore behaviour that is known or likely to result in death, we do not pretend it is not happening, and neither do we avoid asking if we feel it is necessary for an understanding of the client.

In July 2019, it was announced that the 2018 figure for drug-related deaths in Scotland had soared to 1187, 27 per cent higher than in 2017, and the highest since records began in 1996. This exceeds alcohol-related deaths (1136 in 2018), and this rate is nearly three times higher than that of the UK as a whole (Estonia is the second highest) (BBC News 2019). At the Dunes Rehab Center in New York,[5] Shiatsu is being

---

5   https://theduneseasthampton.com/addiction-blog/how-shiatsu-massage-helps-in-addiction-recovery

used in drug and alcohol rehabilitation. Simple though it may seem to some people to decide to give up smoking, or to change lifestyle or behaviour, it can be argued that no one would choose to do something which threatens their life unless they are either unable to change, or do not want to, perhaps because they do not want to live into old age.

Clients with dangerous hobbies

There are people who choose a pastime that might cause death: certain sports and activities such as mountaineering, skydiving, bungee jumping and abseiling. People prepare and train for these sports, though not always, and they might employ others to minimize the risks (to be there to feed them during a marathon, or change their tyres in a motor sport, for example). The death toll is not high (one in 2317 people who base jump, one in 56,587 for swimming, one in 92,325 for cycling, and so on) (Rules of Sport.com n.d.), whereas smoking kills up to half its users (World Health Organization 2019b), but there is good reason to place them in this category.

NP told me about his mountaineering (in places like the Himalayas) at the start of his first session, because an injury he had sustained was the primary reason for coming. He also said that a colleague had recently died on the rocks, and that many others who did what he did knew someone who had either had a life-threatening fall or perished up there. He spent a lot of time doing this and it was closely related to his job, but he was not getting any younger, and had never had a serious long-term partner. This latter was his longer-term aim. He seemed to be weighing up his enjoyment and interest in participating, with the possibility that it could be a problem if he was in a relationship and had a responsibility towards someone else.

This was many years ago and I remember being astonished that he put himself in such danger when he knew what might happen. At the same time, I treated one woman who jumped out of aeroplanes, and a man who had gone over his bicycle handlebars and broken his collarbone for the fourth time, but never thought about giving up high-speed cycling.

(We are trained to notice when clients arrive in a sort of group like this, and so I did ask myself whether there was something I could learn from these risk-taking clients. At the time, I was spending most of my time at home with small children and could only dream of high peaks and deep oceans.)

WB presented with shoulder pain. When Small Intestine arose for the third time, and she was still no better despite her wanting to return to work, I asked if she had ever had an accident and she said no, but her husband had. She had witnessed the very serious vehicle racing accident and the children had also been present. He survived, and after a long time in hospital, a longer recovery at home and a second operation, during which time she had to 'shoulder' all the household tasks and child care, he went back to the sport. She and her bodymind had not forgotten, indeed were still living through some of the trauma. 'I am angry with him for keeping on doing it when we nearly lost him,' she said.

There are many other pursuits in which our clients are involved in taking risks – a sample of those I have worked with over the years includes clients who have taken part in fire-eating, the circus trapeze and dance theatre. I trained as a dancer and I am aware that a certain pride is taken by ballerinas in continuing to dance despite injuries. Putting yourself in danger is also a feature of much performance art: in 1974 Marina Abramović performed Rhythm O, in which articles and instruments which could be used to instil pain and torture were placed on a table beside her. The performer stood impassively while members of the public who attended the show used them on her (Abramović 2013). Whether for thrill, continuing a habit of living life 'on a knife edge', or other reasons, the people who participate in such activities put their lives second to the sport, art or earning money, and this is all part of the client's diagnosis.

Relatives of clients who have had a violent and sudden death

This category of clients includes those who are related to people who have been murdered at home, school and in other public places, by terrorists or perhaps by people who are known to them and/or were already under threat, and those who died in their line of work. Each will have their own characteristics – some totally unexpected, resulting in a degree of unreality, and all probably with intense and extended grief.

The Shiatsu session slows and focuses, supporting the client to stay with reality, however painful, and to creatively problem-solve with ways to move on when the time is right.

There are other situations, ranging from the families of suicide bombers to those who have witnessed or, unwittingly, caused death.

BM was a social worker whose job was to deal with the children involved in an alleged child sex abuse ring. She was having to testify in court when she came for Shiatsu, and her distress was palpable the minute she walked in the room. The first sessions were focused on calming and breathing so she could manage to get through the days. Later, the more in-depth processing started and her emotions were raw. Rare though these incidents are, Shiatsu practitioners may meet such clientele in support centres, as well as in private practice.

Being a serving soldier or soldier's relative means that death is a constant, and someone who has served as a soldier is more likely to commit suicide. Other service personnel, such as police officers, firefighters and ambulance drivers, are often considered to be 'on the frontline' of community violence, possibly dealing with or training to manage terrorist attacks, football crowd problems and gang deaths. Clients' diagnoses may reflect their state of constant alertness and anticipation, and worry over actions taken.

PP served as a fireman more than ten years ago. He reported that every working day he dealt with people or animals in danger, or with managing situations to avoid that. He said he felt as alert on his days off as he was when he was working, and could be called in to support colleagues or fill in where there were shortages, so he did not sleep through the night unless he had had a lot of alcohol during the day. Counselling was available, but he told me,

'No one does it, I don't think. I certainly don't, in case the chief finds out.' His adrenal system was on high alert and he displayed a fighting spirit, with a Liver Jitsu, Kidney Kyo Hara diagnosis at the first session. Initially, it was vital to meet that energy using rotations and stretches. Once the pent-up Ki had dispersed, back palming in time with breathing and firm work on the soles of the feet started to put him in touch with his underlying exhaustion.

Clients who work in dangerous professions

Meg Gaertner-Webster (2019) shares her experience of treating members of the emergency services, including ambulance crew, lifeboat and coastguard crew, firefighters and their families.

Many of the people involved in emergency services are constantly being exposed to the threat to their own lives... What impact does this have on the bms (body, mind, spirit)? In my experience, those who have risked their lives for others are very often affected by their encounters, resulting in deep trauma which may not be apparent until much later, and manifesting as flash backs, sleeplessness, anxiety, over-consumption of alcohol, physical pain and symptoms commonly associated with stress, for example high blood pressure. The chemical effects on the body can be understood when we consider the production of adrenalin and the after effects. Because of the nature of their jobs, these people just have to move on to the next event without time for the previous situation to be processed. If the person is subjected to further risk and to seeing more deaths, they may become desensitized to their feelings in order to cope. While the notion of de-briefing and counselling for the crews is normal in some of the emergency services, little of it ever takes place.

Clients from this group often display spinal pain, headaches, digestive and elimination difficulties. Some of these conditions may be attributed to the physicality of their work, irregular diet, sleeping patterns and working rotas. As a practitioner working with anyone who has trauma, it is especially useful to pay gentle attention to the areas which are not 'talking' to you. There may be many 'false' indicators which offer the client protection in the short term: the sore back is often the cover for a much deeper need. The hard carapace of the being is there for a reason and should not be subjected to hard sedation. It may be useful to consider that these clients trust their lives to the crew/team they work with on a regular basis, and it will take time for the practitioner to become integrated into that person's 'crew'.

As for the families, Meg explains, 'When workers from the emergency services go out on a call or on shift, their families know the risks involved, and often have to be witnesses to their partner's trauma when they return home. The underlying stress level placed on families can, therefore, be quite considerable.'

Clients affected by the media, and friends dying

There are news items about cancer risks and death most days, and many of us know people who have a life-threatening illness or who have died recently. It is, therefore, not surprising that some of our clients are living with high anxiety levels about the possibility of dying. Some of them will have had tests and spent time visiting the doctor, reading on the internet or talking about it a lot with friends, despite the fact that they are told they are well or not in a high-risk category. If it is not themselves who they think will die, it may be their family. They feel that death is nearby, and that is damaging their quality of life and peace of mind. The medical doctor can reassure through testing, prescribe antidepressants or put them on a waiting list for cognitive behavioural therapy or a mindfulness course.

These fears are real, and reassurance does not always help. It is the underlying reason for the fear which is most important, and the root of it is often in other encounters clients have had with death: perhaps a close friend in similar circumstances died and they are still reeling from that, or if they are older, they may be often attending funerals as their friends and acquaintances are dying around them. Terrorism is very much spoken about, and governments spend much money and take elaborate precautions that can highlight the topic even more. There are stabbings and school shootings in unexpected places, so even though there is no war happening in Australia, the US and the UK, we are often reminded of our mortality.

Shiatsu practitioners can usually help. We spend time listening, we take our clients' fears seriously, we have a wide range of possible treatment strategies, we can support our clients to relax and express their feelings, and there are even specific acupoints (Shu Mansion

(Shufu KD 27), for example) and meridians (BL) that deal directly with fear of death.

Mental health, medication and state of mind
Mental health sector

The most common sector in which Shiatsu practitioners have been employed in the UK is mental health. Clients in this setting may have attempted suicide or be facing death as a result of extreme behaviour. They could have caused others' deaths, if it is a prison hospital, although it must be noted that a very low proportion of violent crimes are committed by those with mental health issues (Time to Change 2019). This environment poses different challenges. It includes those with Western medical diagnoses of psychosis, schizophrenia, clinical depression, anxiety and mania, as well as those who have self-harmed, are delusional or drug and alcohol dependent. It is to such institutions that those who are 'a risk to themselves' or 'a risk to others' are referred, sectioned or self-admitted. It is likely that psychological loss is involved in almost all cases.

Katharine Hall (2010, p.6), a Shiatsu practitioner, writes:

> Working with people who do not want to be in hospital in the first place, and do not necessarily agree that they are unwell, is certainly different. The majority of patients I see are sectioned under the Mental Health Act (as a risk to themselves or others). The involuntary aspect of people's hospitalization is a huge contrast to working with people in private practice... The innately fragile, vulnerable states that many patients are in...can be exacerbated by being locked up with other distressed individuals... Many of the problems that clients present will spring from ancestral, environmental, economic and social causes aggravated by unhealthy lifestyle and nutrition.

While there has been some employment of Shiatsu practitioners in psychiatric hospitals in the UK over the years (a number of Shiatsu practitioners have worked at the Maudsley in South East England, and practitioners have volunteered in other places such as the Royal Edinburgh Psychiatric Hospital in Edinburgh, Scotland), complementary and alternative therapies are not typically available through the National Health Service as a treatment for mental health problems. This is because they are not recognized as evidence-based treatment options by the National Institute for Health and Care Excellence (NICE) – the organization that aims to produce guidelines on best practice in healthcare.

Due to the nature of mental health institutions, all patients will be under the care of a team involving the patient and his family. Although it is necessary for everyone to work as closely as possible together in order to provide the best for them, it must be remembered that Shiatsu practitioners are likely to be the only ones addressing the whole person, and therefore have a lot to offer. Rather than focusing on one body system or sticking with a particular medical diagnosis, it is the Shiatsu practitioner who holds the whole bodymind, and it is they who can be aware of complications before they arise or who can give the client the sense of being an entire human being who is not defined by their disease. (This is unique and consequently a message to be promoted in the future.)

In the UK, traditional medical treatment is reliant on talk therapy (principally psychiatry and also psychotherapy in the form of cognitive behavioural therapy); drug therapy (medication); electro-convulsive treatment; and, in rare cases in the UK, neurosurgery for mental disorder, which is also listed in the US in addition to repetitive transcranial magnetic stimulation, deep brain stimulation and vagus nerve stimulation. It is the *Diagnostic and Statistical Manual of Mental Disorders* (*DSM-5*), published by the American Psychiatric Association (2013), that is used to make an accurate diagnosis.

This array of procedures, medication levels and multiple psychological diagnoses together with Shiatsu results in complicated outcomes. It can therefore be hard, and it may be unnecessary, to know whether it was Shiatsu or another aspect of treatment that was responsible for any benefit or worsening of a patient's condition.

Depression, grief and clinical depression

In 2017, more than one in eight Americans aged 12–25 experienced a major depressive episode, according to the National Institute of Mental Health (2019).

Like all conditions, depression has a scale of seriousness and variation. At one end, we are working with clients who experience low moods that come and go; then there are those who are weary, unjoyful and trudge through life; and at the other end of the scale are people who cannot get out of bed, wash or look after their children, for whom the depression is unremitting. In some cases, there will be a desire for relief from the chronic or repetitive symptoms through death; many of those who commit suicide have a diagnosis of clinical depression. It is important to note that people who have experienced severe depression and found relief are extremely scared that it might start again and are therefore loath to stop or reduce medication (which in any case is not a good idea without the help of the physician, and then only gradually).

As these people are often alone for long periods and shun contact, communication can be a lifeline for those with depression. Finding a balance between being listened to and being involved in something else, such as looking after a plant or an animal, or supporting a charitable cause, can be useful. There are a number of challenges in working with chronically depressed clients:

- Will they attend Shiatsu regularly, particularly when the depression is at its worst? Making the next appointment at the end of the previous session is always worthwhile, although there is a higher than average risk of no-show. In these cases, contacting them to ask for a cancellation fee may be a good excuse to communicate, but it may also mean that the client with already low self-esteem is hurt.

- Can you tell where the line is drawn between being very low, and being suicidal and in need of medical attention? Make sure that the client is under medical care and make a note that you have recommended that they see a doctor, even if they refuse or you fear that they may not. You might even feel the need to get them to sign a statement saying you have advised this, to protect yourself in the worst-case scenario.

The difference between grief and depression

It is important to be able to distinguish between a natural response to grief and depression. Many of the symptoms are the same, such as not finding enjoyment as you have in the past, and feeling hopeless. There is or has been a trend towards offering antidepressants to those who are grieving, when their state of mind, though desperate at the loss, is normal and will pass with the right amount of understanding and support.

For those who live alone or have sequestered themselves even though they would prefer to be with others, and are facing death, the Shiatsu practitioner can be a vital connection. These clients can be any age, though more likely to be elderly. They are coping with multiple aspects of life: managing to feed themselves and provide a roof over their own heads, as well as managing their various symptoms and being closer to death. You might have met the client in your neighbourhood or often seen them at the shops. Your role may be a hybrid of community supporter and Shiatsu practitioner (as long as they are able to actively choose to have the treatments). You may be offering the treatments for free, and boundaries might be elastic, but you could be a rare contact and certainly one of the only people who touches the person in this specific way. Some will be embroiled in loss, and others will seem to be clear of it.

CW contacted me himself to ask for treatments. He was 78 when he first came and clearly was not able or interested in keeping himself and his clothes clean. He had a wide range of physical symptoms and was sure that he would die soon, which he anticipated as a relief. He said he often did not get out of bed for days, 'so when I go they'll know where to find me'. The Shiatsu helped his cough, making him more able to lie down to sleep. He was strong, and over time his body did not deteriorate much, but he either developed or revealed some mental health issues, becoming extremely angry and abusive more than once. I ascertained that he was on a social work list and in receipt of a meal delivery service, which made me feel slightly reassured when the time came (after a year and a half) to stop seeing him on account of his behaviour. With his permission, I wrote to his doctor to explain that he had been coming to me and that it was now no longer appropriate.

Medication and state of mind

Many Shiatsu clients are on medication. This can affect Shiatsu diagnosis and treatment. Valium sedates and suppresses the Liver Yang. The reappearance of a major symptom is a common side effect, and the Shiatsu therapist who touches someone taking an antidepressant often senses a blandness and a lack of responsive Ki. The aim of these medications is both to manage the disease and keep the patient alive.

There is a general assumption that everyone wants to continue living, but this may not be so once we look under the surface, or at least it may be more complicated than that.

UD knew the woman who committed suicide by jumping out of a window quite well. He did not know much about her mental illness before it happened, but had been upset by her writing him an angry letter shortly before she died, and even asked his wife to choose between them, causing a great deal of pain and difficulty. Later they were told that she had been on suicide watch with her father in the next room just before the time of death. The family believed that she had been on the wrong medication and that it had made things worse or caused delusions (and might have explained the out-of-character behaviour over the letter). After she died, he reported thinking he had seen her often, glimpsing her out of the corner of his eye or seeing her disappear around a corner in the city where they had lived. It lasted for 6–12 months.

The Shiatsu offered a quiet place for UD to focus on his complicated feelings. Through the grounding touch (Spleen Jitsu) he said he recognized that nothing could now be done, no more amends could be made, and that he would never know if the effort he had gone to before the suicide to heal the situation was successful or not. He gestured to his back (Bladder was Kyo in the Hara diagnosis) when he told me that he felt he had contributed to her pain or even her death. I repeated his phrase, 'You feel that you contributed to her pain, even her death', which was followed by a silence. He was in supine and I was holding on to his heels and leaning back (both engaging the Bladder and encouraging the Ki downwards) when he said that he had been reading that things can get out of proportion if you have a mental illness, that it can sometimes be a reaction to the medication. After the session ended, he said, 'So, maybe, her suicide was not caused by me or anyone else.'

Mental health and abuse

There is a recognized connection between mental health issues and abuse:

> It is now well accepted that abuse (both in childhood and in adult life) is often the main factor in the development of depression, anxiety and other mental health disorders, and may lead to sleep disturbances, self-harm, suicide and attempted suicide, eating disorders and substance misuse. (Women's Aid Federation of England 2015)

Shiatsu will usually address the underlying cause while attempting to stabilize the presenting symptoms. In such cases, the practitioner must not act alone, but alongside other health professionals. What we can offer, which they cannot, is an awareness of self-esteem matters, and ways to touch that will bring the client into a deep contact with their own sense of themselves, and our ability to identify causal factors.

Psychotic illness and death

Those with psychotic illnesses are likely to be scared, according to findings by the Victoria State Government (2018): 'A sizeable group of Australians with a psychotic illness [for example, schizophrenia] reported that they had experienced physical abuse within the previous year.' For instance:

- 18 per cent had been a victim of violence.
- 17 per cent attempted suicide or deliberate self-harm.
- 15 per cent did not feel safe in their neighbourhood area.

This shows that people with a psychotic illness carry the added burden of feeling vulnerable to harm and therefore death.

Suicide and assisted suicide
Suicide

In 2016, suicide was the tenth leading cause of death in the US and the second among 10–34-year-olds (National Institute of Mental Health 2017). 'From 1985 onwards, external factors, such as drug misuse, suicide and self-harm, were the leading cause of death for young people, affecting more men than women' (Office for National Statistics 2017).

Women make more attempts than men, and men are more likely to succeed. People aged 45–64 have the highest suicide rate, and people who do this are likely to be single and living in rural areas. In the US, there are 25 attempts for every suicide (Today on YouTube 2018). People identifying as LGBTQ, especially if they live in countries where their human rights are not respected or there is the threat of death, also sadly feature in the statistics. Ninety per cent of people who commit suicide in the UK are experiencing mental distress (Time to Change 2019).

Suicidal ideation (the term used for someone who wants to take their own life or is thinking about it) must be taken seriously. There are two sorts: active and passive. Passive suggests they wish to commit suicide, but have no plans to do so; active that they not only wish to, but also intend to and are therefore planning it. It is thought that 80 per cent of suicides happen without much forethought, but at the same time it is vital that we know the warning signs. However many times you hear someone say that it was unexpected, the person has usually spoken about it, been to see their doctor (about something physical), and offered other hints.

People may come to us if they know that we provide a safe environment and are open and accepting in our manner. We are also likely to recognize the signs, because we take a full and comprehensive case history that covers all four levels of the bodymind.

Useful questions to ask the client:

- Have you been to the doctor?

- Have you ever attempted or thought about suicide? (If they reply, 'Oh no, it's not that bad', you are probably safe to work with them.)

- Do you have someone at home to support you?

- Are you taking medication, and if so, what sort?

We are trained to pick up the signs:

- This client is behaving significantly differently from others.

- You get a feeling, a hunch. Take it seriously!

- You notice incongruities – things do not seem to add up.

The recognized indications that someone is at risk of suicide:

- Talk of suicide – imagining being dead, of dying while asleep, of having an accident and dying.

- Alcohol and substance abuse.

- Psychomotor agitation – pacing, tapping, movements with no point to them.

- Lack of concentration, forgetting appointments and not caring.

- No pleasure in usually pleasurable things, for example a new baby in the family.

- Making a will, giving away possessions, saying 'goodbye'.

- Risk taking, for example unprotected sex; impaired judgement (the client says something is fine when you know it is not; for example, he reports that someone hit him, but says it was okay).

- Mood swings – anger, irritability, rage, impulsivity.

- Unremitting grief.

- Buying a firearm (in the US) – it is ten times more likely that a suicide happens in a home where a gun is owned. In 1996 in Australia and the UK (the year of the Dunblane shootings), owning firearms became severely restricted with significant positive results.

- Buying lots of pills.

- Researching suicide on the internet.

Triggers:

- Chronic pain or illness.

- Diagnoses of depression, bipolar disorder, brain injury.

- Guilt.

- Anxiety, panic.

- Loneliness and isolation (not married, no children living at home).

- Low self-esteem and self-worth, self-hate, self-criticism, self-anger.

- Irregularity of lifestyle – missing meals, working late at night.

- Hopelessness, helplessness.

- Insomnia, lethargy.

- Eating disorder.

- Significant loss.

We are always seeking an amalgamation or pattern of symptoms in order for us to distinguish between one diagnosis and treatment plan and another.

Situations known to have caused suicide:

- Relationship breakdown.

- Work/exam 'failure' or pressure.

- Financial worries.

- Abuse.

- Trauma.

- Post-traumatic stress disorder.

- Family history of suicide.

Note: A client who is on antidepressants is not necessarily suicidal. If there is a sudden change and she has become happy, however, there could be a variety of reasons, one of which is the possibility that she has decided to act on her thoughts and has a suicide plan.

The Shiatsu Society's (UK) (n.d.) *Code of Conduct and Ethics* states that there may be situations in which a client tells you about suicidal thoughts or attempts. In situations such as this, it suggests, you should inform their general practitioner (GP), and wherever possible, in advance, you should seek the consent of the client to disclose the information in that way. If you do not have their GP's details, then phone a medical helpline, your own doctor for advice, or even the hospital emergency department. If you think they are at immediate risk, stay with them and contact a friend or relative who can accompany them and make the decision.

If a client commits suicide, the consequences may be very challenging, ranging from your own sadness at not having been able to help (if someone is determined, then they will find a way to end their own life), to a relative accusing you of being complicit in some way.

If you do report it to the doctor, then the client may find themselves on suicide watch and be resentful. Whatever happens, you will need support, whether from your colleagues or supervisor.

If someone (more often it is likely to be a woman, but not always) talks about an abusive partner and is obviously feeling helpless, she must be taken seriously. The number of women being killed by their partner (because of jealousy, power, anger and rage, alcohol and so on) is high.

If you think your client might be suicidal or if he said he was when you saw him at the previous session, do broach the subject. This advice is backed up by professionals in the field. Asking the question directly and openly shows that you care. Do not imagine it will go away – very often the client feels he cannot speak about it, and if he cannot or does not talk about it, it may get worse.

Not long after graduating, I was standing up on a crowded bus when a young corporate client from a local business whom I had not seen for a while said hello. She told me, there among all the commuters, that she had been off work for a while because she had attempted suicide. I could not remember her being an at-risk client and was horrified to hear her news. After giving me some details in a rather off-hand way, she jauntily said goodbye and got off at the next stop. I can only hope that her message was that she was well now, but nevertheless it is unusual to divulge such information in such a way, and I would have made private contact with her afterwards if I had had her details.

She left me with the information – perhaps it was a burden off her shoulders – and all I could do was send my best wishes through the ether. This wayward, Fire behaviour is not untypical of one type of suicidal client – slightly hysterical, a lack of boundaries and an impetuous need to talk. Later I learned how to close part of myself off before I left the treatment room so that I did not pick up others' vibes, nor give the impression that I was always in therapist mode and thus ready to listen in unexpected places.

If you would like to make a recommendation at the end of the Shiatsu, the sorts of things which are recognized as having helped people who have attempted suicide are music, exercise, including walking in the fresh air and dancing, meditation or other sort of activity to learn to control the mind, cognitive behavioural therapy and other forms of psychotherapy, being with friends and family who love them, learning something new, caring for a dog, doing things for other people, being in nature and belief in some sort of spirituality or God. As with all recommendations, make sure that you use them sparingly, choose wisely so that the one you select is appropriate and manageable, agree with the client why you are making it, and check later whether they have tried it and with what results, so you can change it if need be.

Some clients report that they would like to commit suicide, would prefer to be dead, but that they are staying alive because of someone else who needs them. This is serious and should be followed up in some way.

Whatever the age, there is a particular danger of a client committing suicide soon after someone very close to them has died in that way, be it a best friend, partner or family member.

AC felt totally overwhelmed after her partner's suicide and said she could not imagine surviving without him, even though the children were so young. The responsibility, she said, was unbearable, and she felt so alone with them. As practitioners, we must particularly look out for our clients at a time when they are so very vulnerable. Make sure they have added support, and, if the thought occurs to you, ask them if they are in any danger of doing the same.

There are occasionally stories in the media about famous people committing suicide, and there are known cases in which someone who has heard them then copies their behaviour. Usually this is only if they already have other triggers or emotions. Young people, or those who share very strong feelings with someone else, for example religious beliefs, are more susceptible than others. If it was someone they admired, or who was unwittingly glorified, if the client is in their teens or twenties, when political activism can be prompted by strong feelings of alienation or identification with a cause (and they are already feeling misunderstood or hounded for what they believe in), or if they self-identify, then they may be at risk.

The Crisis Centre (2013) in Vancouver, Canada, states:

We know that those at risk for suicide do not necessarily want to die, but do want help in reducing the pain they are experiencing so that they can go on to lead productive, fulfilling lives… At some level, all suicide attempts are cries for help by individuals experiencing a high degree of desperation.

It can happen, after years of mental health issues, that someone attempts suicide. In one case, a student's father started to express suicidal thoughts after multiple failed attempts by her mother. As a result, she was later diagnosed with post-traumatic stress disorder, which she acknowledged later had been the case for a long time (Jenkins 2019).

You may have strong feelings about this, especially if you have been personally influenced by suicide. There is a debate about whether ending one's life is an act of ultimate self-determination or an unforgivable burden for loved ones. Giving Shiatsu to someone whose relative or friend has committed suicide will be a matter of supporting them through shock and grief, complex and desperate emotions, perhaps including self-blame if they feel they should have noticed or stopped the person, and possible difficulties because of their spiritual beliefs if suicide is forbidden (as it is in the Islamic faith, for example).

Euthanasia and doctor-assisted suicide

Rod MacLeod and colleagues (2012) cite several different interpretations and definitions to assisted suicide. It is a complicated issue, and if there is any chance that you will be asked to assist or even comment on euthanasia and doctor-assisted suicide, then I suggest that you inform yourself of the up-to-date situation (it changes often as legislation changes in different countries). Briefly, a doctor who is allowed by law to end someone's life by painless means, as long as the patient and their family agrees, is practising euthanasia. Note that there is active and passive, as well as voluntary and involuntary, euthanasia, depending on who gives permission and whether the patient is conscious or not. For example, a doctor who helps someone commit suicide if they ask him, by providing a lethal dose for self-administration, is performing doctor-assisted suicide. Active euthanasia is more controversial, and it is more likely to involve religious, moral, ethical and compassionate arguments.

Voluntary euthanasia is currently legal in Belgium, Luxembourg,

Colombia and the Netherlands. Switzerland, Germany, Japan, Canada and certain states of the US allow assisted suicide.

Clients with different faiths and cultural traditions

There are many reasons why knowing about death practices and beliefs from different cultures and religions is important for our client work. We aim to be inclusive and open-minded. Each client will have values derived from a specific religion or practice, or a wide range of other sources. It has been shown that when facing death, many of us either revert to an original, childhood or family custom, give it up entirely, or begin to follow a new way, and this spiritual aspect will certainly be present when working with clients who are facing death. We have the right to say 'no' to giving Shiatsu, but it should not be on the grounds of race, creed or colour, unless we feel threatened or in danger because of their statements or behaviour.

Shiatsu practitioners who aim to work where there is a cross-section of the community, such as in a hospice, will be well advised to know some basics in this respect.

Putting aside our own beliefs allows us to focus on the client's during the session. Their values will tell us about that person's attitude and are therefore part of the diagnosis, the overall picture of the client. We may then ascertain the level on which it is useful for us to work. Many are comforted by knowing that their relatives will go to heaven or somewhere beautiful (often the place is a garden (Eden) or a reed bed), where they will be with others who have previously died. If their faith holds strong, they are unafraid, because they know what will happen to them; they will not need us to support their spiritual aspect. For example, when working with a Sikh you will usually find that there is a peaceful and accepting energy at the end because they believe in the transmigration of the soul, that it never dies. They celebrate because the soul has the chance to meet the Wondrous Giver of Knowledge, Waheguru, and it is unlikely that they will be distressed (Singh 2019).

We can learn so much from each other about what might happen after death, where we go and why. This is usually clearly laid out in both organized religion and the tenets of non-religious groups. If we are unsure or question what will happen to us when the time comes for our own death, what a privilege it is to get insight into what another person's beliefs rest on, what drives and sustains them.

The Aboriginals, the original peoples of Australia, believe that, after death, the new situation is not too different from the person's earthly life in which he or she had many roles. One part of the deceased may move to the *Land of the Dead*, often named the *sky-world*, and as long as certain rituals were carried out during their life and at their death they will be very well there. Alternatively, the dead person might return to the site where spirit children await rebirth, or merge with the great ancestral and creative beings. This explains why the Aboriginals are very protective of places they call sacred – it is the location for what remains of a deceased member of their community. Like Catholics, Aboriginal people believe in resurrection, that spirits are resurrected into living beings (Monroe 2010).

Theosophists believe in Summerland (also called the astral plane), depicted as a place where souls who have been good in their previous lives go between incarnations. They believe the Summerlands are maintained by hosts of planetary angels serving Sanat Kumara, who is the governing deity and leader of the Spiritual Hierarchy of Earth. Sanat Kumara is believed to rule over our planet from the floating city of Shamballa, existing on the etheric plane (between the physical plane and the astral plane), about five miles (eight km) above the Gobi Desert (Leadbeater 2007). 'The final, permanent and eternal afterlife to which Theosophists believe most people will go millions or billions of years in the future, after our cycle of reincarnations in this round is over, is called Nirvana, and is located beyond this physical cosmos' (Wikipedia 2019c).

Like theosophists, many people believe that they will be judged before being assigned a place after death. This is important for the Shiatsu practitioner to know, because clients can be under a great deal of pressure to follow the rules in case they go to hell or are found wanting. Even if they break with their former traditions, anyone who was raised by parents or others who instilled this in them at an early age will still find it hard to shake off. Like all early learning, it can find its way into unconscious behaviour, and Shiatsu may be chosen to manage this. The awareness-raising aspect to what we do is useful as a first step, but only at the specific request of the client.

Other religions recognize many gods and goddesses, like Shinto, the world's fifth largest religion. This open attitude means that they can add in other beliefs and practices without fear of being damned (eCondolence.com n.d.).

In Ancient Greece, heroic or great deeds were believed to be the only way the dead could move onwards and forwards to a bountiful location. Admission to the Elysian Fields (Wikipedia 2019a) was initially reserved for mortals related to the gods and other heroes, but later the list of possible candidates was lengthened to include the righteous or chosen ones, making it particularly hard to know if that included you or not. Though this is historical (or literary), it results in worshippers eternally striving, as they do not know exactly what will constitute *good enough*. This behaviour is shared by many religious followers (Catholics and the Church of England, for example). For some, this offers a structure and a reason for living; for others, it feels as if they are lacking in personal choice. Hindus believe in *karma* and are therefore aware that bad deeds will transform into negative merit (BBC 2019).

There are those who long for the end because they know they will be in paradise (Islam), and those who fear hell (hadephobia): the Christian Bible is full of descriptions such as 'a place of consuming worms and undying fire' (Mark 9:48), and warnings of pits of fire.

Some of our clients will be very connected with the cycles of life and death through regular rituals (Wiccan, for example), and others will feel disconnected and free-falling, either searching for meaning or resolved that there is none.

After death – mourning

Mourning is an old word. It is often associated with the outward expression of the internal response, which is grief. A period of mourning is the time allocated to remembering and showing others that this is happening. Mourning is also a term for the black clothes worn at the funeral in the West (and Japan), and after someone's death to show that they are grieving. As we know, white is the colour associated with death in China. It symbolizes purity of spirit at a time when the Po and Hun separate (see Chapter 2). It is also white in India, whereas red has been worn at South African funerals, and purple in Thailand (Funeral Guide 2017).

Display of mourning

Mourning can last for different amounts of time, and it can be useful for others to know this in order to continue to support and offer understanding. In Papua New Guinea, the women who are mourning their husbands scrape grey pigment from stones and make necklaces of seeds coloured with it. They take these seeds off, one by one, as the period of mourning passes (around nine months); thus it is clear how long ago the men died by the number still hanging around the women's necks (Funeral Guide 2017).

Jewish communities observe various rituals during the mourning period, including kriah, the rending or tearing of clothes or black cloth which is then displayed for 7–30 days (My Jewish Learning n.d.).

It is unlikely that anyone in Britain today places a crepe and ribbon badge over the front door knocker as they did in Victorian times (Langford 2014), whereas in China, it is seven days after the death when the spirit is believed to return home, so to ensure that it does not get lost, the family will place a red plaque outside their home (T-Knox 2019). There are still some outward signs of bereavement in the West: black armbands are sometimes worn by sports players when a team member dies; those who wear badges (firefighters, police officers) may place black mourning bands around them in remembrance; and members of the public wore black loops of ribbon when Princess Diana died in 1997 and was buried in the UK.

If you are working with a mourning client, the Shiatsu itself can play a part of that function, particularly if they cannot attend the funeral or are at odds with the service or procedure that has been chosen by others.

Funeral ceremony/procession

The funeral ceremony or procession is a worldwide ritual used to mark a death. An opportunity for relatives and friends to pay tribute and mourn together, it is a necessary part of many clients' religious practices. If relevant to those involved and/or the deceased, it also serves as a rite of passage, marking the time when those living give the body over to God or the spirits for safe-keeping on the journey to the next life or the hereafter.

In the streets of Muslim countries, a funeral procession is a familiar sight and it is expected that the mourning women will wail and keen for all to hear, although men are generally silent and stoical. Sometimes professional mourners are employed. Buddhists, Hindus, Jews, Orthodox Greeks and Russians all have their own traditions, and with those rituals come different approaches to acknowledging and talking about death. We may meet clients from all of these backgrounds, so it is useful for us to become familiar with their particular types of ritual.

In countries where Protestantism has not been the historical context for government and monarchy, death plays a more visible part, a different role in life, and is embraced in other ways. Whereas those attending a Protestant funeral may stand quietly and conceal their tears if at all possible, in Catholic countries there is the tradition of the Day of the Dead, where parties of people visit the cemetery to publicly mourn. These rituals signify a relationship with the end of life that is unfamiliar to some, but, perhaps, familiarizes the mourners with death and the sight of a dead body at an earlier stage of life.

The wake

A wake is a social gathering, traditionally held before a funeral, in the house of the deceased and with the body present.

In Japan, the funeral is held as soon as possible after death.

> A Japanese wake is called *tsuya*, literally *passing the night*, and relatives moisten the dying or deceased person's lips with water, a practice known as *water of the last moment*. Most Japanese homes maintain Buddhist altars, or *butsudan*, for use in Buddhist ceremonies; some also have Shinto shrines, as no one religion prevails. When a death occurs, the shrine is closed and covered with white paper to keep out the impure spirits of the dead, a custom called *kamidana-fūji*. A small table decorated with flowers, and incense and a candle is placed next to the deceased's bed. (Wikipedia 2019b)

Catholics also have a tradition of the wake. It allows for the family and friends to have one more opportunity to pray and express their feelings, sometimes publicly, to remember and to say goodbye. It might last for a few days or take place on the evening before the Rite of Committal, known as the Vigil.

YH's brother died very suddenly on the kitchen floor while getting breakfast for his young children, and he was reeling from the suddenness of the tragedy. The couple were primary school teachers at different rural schools in Ireland, and they held a traditional Irish wake with an open coffin that stood on legs in the parlour. Both schools shut for the day and mourners were taken in buses to pay their respects. The environment, my client reported, was positive and upbeat; the children ran under and around the casket while the adults drank tea and whiskey and ate sandwiches. It made death very much part of life, and there was no taboo about crying, laughing and remembering the deceased. Private grieving started only after everyone had gone home and left the family to themselves to begin acclimatizing to life without their loved one. When my client returned home, he was at a distance from the rest of his relatives and life had changed, particularly because of a new fear of losing his own partner and child.

Burial rituals

The Chinese believe that certain rituals must be fulfilled in order that their dead are appeased. 'Han burial customs provided nourishment and comfort for the Po with the placement of grave goods, including food, commodities, and even money within the tomb of the deceased' (Hansen 2000, p.119). Many religions, such as Sikhism and Christianity, bathe and dress the deceased, although the Sikh relatives must leave the Articles of Faith with the person and not shave their hair.

Clients in the UK, US or Australia, especially those whose relatives hail from the Asian subcontinent, may feel that intensive death rituals which are part of their inherited traditions are onerous. They may feel an internal conflict between those duties and the necessities of their daily lives, beliefs or lack of them. Shiatsu can help those clients connect with their true feelings, either to discover the strength they need to follow and honour what their parents expect, or to be able to identify an alternative, personal way.

> 'Out beyond ideas of wrongdoing and right doing there is a field. I'll meet you there.' Rumi

The grave

In keeping with Japanese custom, the dead often receive Buddhist names, which are engraved on their headstones. Once delivered from this world, they move on to the next, as Buddhas themselves. That way, they will not mistakenly return to this world if the living happen to call them by their old names. In fact, tradition is changing, and a non-religious name is sometimes being chosen instead, something from nature.

Celebration

On the Mexican holiday (also) known as the *Day of the Dead* (*el Día de los Muertos*) (2018), families welcome back the souls of their deceased relatives for a brief reunion that includes food, drink and celebration. All over the Catholic world, on 2 November, people go to cemeteries and churches with flowers and candles to offer prayers in a life-affirming ceremony to honour their dead. It serves both as an opportunity to remember and also to celebrate.

Rite and ritual

With its Japanese and Chinese origins, Shiatsu has inherited a relationship with ritual. We might use it to prepare for our work or directly with an individual or group. We may participate in a Fire Walk or a Sweat Lodge, a solstice or a Humanist naming ceremony as part of developing our own energy. If ritual is a normal part of our practice, then the clients we have attracted will accept it as part of the session, and when we are working with loss it can then be extended to play a larger role if necessary. While some of the people we work with will not be interested or will have their own traditions, others will appreciate the chance to remember and release their emotions when the time is right, and find it comforting.

A ritual is a ceremony that progresses over time, performed regularly or as a one-off, especially devised for a particular reason or occasion and with a specific meaning. It can be an aid to recovery from death, support the grieving process or be an integral part of the mourning period.

The Shinto religion, practised by nearly 80 per cent of the Japanese population, seems to ground its followers in the past. Old traditions are honoured: family members are remembered, times of the year are marked, and historical events are celebrated, enabling people to share and connect with each other. Rituals focused on the transition from life to death, or a life with someone and a life without, can be a valuable way to mark the event.

Shiatsu fulfils many of these aspects. Some practitioners stress them more than others:

- Wearing specific clothes, often all white or black.

- Bowing, to show respect and thank the client, guiding spirits.

- Following a certain protocol each time.

- Always using certain words or phrases – 'This will happen first, then this. How does it feel?' Repeating the client's words back to them.

- Using similar movements each time – diagnosis, observing a routine around the body, working the Kyo and then the Jitsu meridians.

- Decorating/scenting the room with essential oils or incense.

- Using a more Japanese style – entering the *dojo* with a bow, honouring your teachers, taking your shoes off, making or pouring water or tea.

- Having an altar of some sort in the room, or a Buddha, or a picture of a Master, using a token, a representation of an animal, a stone or a shell.

- Including a prayer or mantra, chanting or gesturing.

Almost all of us set an aim, follow some sort of pattern (prepare, meet, greet, touch, say goodbye and so on), and follow in the tradition of someone (a teacher, a teacher's teacher). For the client, Shiatsu can be a ritual of sorts: travelling to the same place, the same practitioner, maybe on the same time of day and week or month, for the same duration for many years, coming back into the body, focusing on themselves. Among the quotes from my clients are: 'The time I tune into myself'; 'a place out of time where I can attend to my soul'; 'an opportunity to be away from life and connect'.

There are those who return to the rite of organized religion when they are near death. It offers a structure in which to focus on what is happening and what is important, and may be familiar from childhood: repeating a liturgy, being invited to confess (with a priest or in silent/led prayer), being offered forgiveness, and believing in heaven or some similar place of rest.

Ritual fulfils the function of connecting us with some sort of lineage, tradition or spiritual practice. It can be a most useful way to acknowledge what we do in the early 21st century, where in the West it is sometimes seen as an alternative to a capitalist way of life, an antidote to spending so much time and energy in making money, or as an alternative to screen time.

Devising a ritual for and with your client

If you think your client would benefit from it, or they have asked you, you could devise a ritual when they are facing death or are at the end of life. While the parameters of ritual are very open, there are some questions you might like to consider:

- Is there a clear intention? (This aligns the Ki.) Is it to mark the loss of someone loved? To help let go during the bereavement period?

- What is the connection to Shiatsu? Consider why you are involved. Will it involve touch by the practitioner, someone else or the client? Is it based on the Five Elements? Is it that you, the practitioner, have experience of this and the client needs a companion or ideas or support in person or planning?

- Will the ritual be instead of a Shiatsu session, or part of it? Have you spoken about payment?

- Is it a one-off or something that the client will repeat? If the latter, will you both make a record of it so they can remember what to do?

- Will the process or effect need evaluating or reviewing at a later date?

- How can you help your client to find a way to discover what he wants? For example, you could use this as the aim of the Shiatsu.

Making an altar

Decide together:

- Why? If this has come from the client then he probably knows, so it is just a matter of clarifying and focusing.

- Where? If at the client's own home, will the discussion take place after Shiatsu (allowing time at the end)? Will the client take notes to aid memory? Or if it will be part of a ritual that will happen in the Shiatsu room or somewhere else altogether, then perhaps an advance planning session will allow everything to be collected and prepared. Choose somewhere that benefits the mood or energy.

- What? The items for placing on the altar will relate to the function – perhaps a photo of, and keepsake from, the deceased, a candle or flower(s), food or drink, a crystal. If in nature, perhaps you will collect things when you are there, so it will take longer. You can be creative in how you curate this.

- If you are using the Five Elements, then you will need a smell, taste, something aural (music, chant or song – you may require equipment), and touch.

- Will you assemble the altar in advance or will doing that be part of the ritual?

- If the altar is being dismantled afterwards, is there a way for the client to carry or transport it home?

Reading, whispering, chanting, storytelling and sounding

As you sit beside someone who is nearing the end of their lives, you may find yourself making sounds other than talking, while or instead of giving more recognizable Shiatsu. The person may be conscious or not, but the way we communicate is through Ki, and Ki encompasses sound as well as touch. Sound touches, or at least it is effective through vibration in the way that touch is. If you use sound, you are part of an age-old tradition from many cultures.

The Sikhs will participate in a devotional reading of the holy scripture at home or in the Gudvara (place of worship) after death, as 'when read with understanding it can provide comfort and consolation to the grieving' (Singh 2019).

Tibetan Buddhists believe that the soul separates from the physical body and moves through levels or *bardos*. In the Tibetan *Book of the Dead* or *Bardo Thodol*, it is explained, 'There are three bardos encapsulating various aspects of the afterlife realm, in which the living whisper instructions of comfort, peace, and guidance to the deceased' (Sipper n.d.).

There are many accounts of Shiatsu practitioners using sound, song or chanting. Rose Fuhrmann writes:

> Some people from my body, voice and breath work group have set up a group for sounding for the very ill and dying. In one session, we did a role play in which one participant was in the role of the dying person (a strong experience in itself!) and the others sounded to her in turn… From my perspective, the most important one was that the person dying as well as the people listening perceived the subtle differences in the approach or motivation or mindset of the sounder. To me, it felt as if some people's sounding was of the nature of calling the person back, not letting them die as it were.[6]

Some Shiatsu practitioners have a tantric practice where repeating mantras and meditating on the various figures of a particular tradition can help develop the qualities they require for their work. Quan Yin, for example, the bodhisattva Avalokiteshvara, is said to be full of compassion, and being with this spirit over time is said to support you in finding those qualities in yourself. If you are working with clients who are familiar with these ideas, bringing them into your sessions is likely to be natural and supportive.

Storytelling

Samhain (All Souls' or All Saints' Day) is part of the pagan religious festival originating from a Celtic tradition. It is the end and the beginning of the year, 'that time when we think of the ancestors, that time when the veil is unusually thin and the Other Realm is palpable' (Tadhg Jonathan 2018). In the past, there would be storytelling time in villages or round camp fires, where tales would be told of spirits crossing over. These folk stories served to pass on the old ways to children and adults who were scared of death or unsure, and instruct their listeners in a deceptively simple manner.

---

6   From a letter to Kate Man, reproduced in the Shiatsu Society helpsheet on death.

Dedication

The client may like to dedicate the Shiatsu to the deceased, or to have a Shiatsu session before attending the funeral for centring and composure. There are different religious practices that follow death. For example, Muslims may wash the body together and then shroud it ready for burial. The Japanese may watch altogether as an *encoffiner* (a professional) washes and prepares the body for cremation.

Memory

Many of the ways and traditions elucidated above are about remembering and keeping the memories alive. As we age, it is sensible to have such rituals, and is a way of sharing.

When I was writing about my father's death, I realized that I could not remember how much time had elapsed between his diagnosis and his death – it was clear that what I thought was true was not so, because the days and months did not add up. There are reasons why we and our clients struggle to remember certain things: age, yes, but also if it is not important, or if it holds emotional distress, in order that it is not disturbing us. We know that in TCM, as the Jing becomes depleted, our short-term memory can go with it, and this affects the balance with the Fire element, as a result of which our long-term memory can sharpen.

Ghosts, angels, spirits, past lives, and psychic activity

Belief in spirits goes back as far as the earliest peoples. Our own Chinese Medicine talks of the Hun; some Buddhists write about people visiting each other in dreams; shamans call on animal spirits; some pagans may believe in nature spirits; spiritualists believe that the spirits of the dead can and do communicate with the living; and, indeed, Christians believe that Jesus came back from the dead and that the Holy Ghost has influence over those who are alive.

Many people who do not align themselves with a religion or spiritual group sense that a dead parent or relative is still with them after they have died. Further, they sense that this spirit may see what they are doing, and even try to send them a message. There are huge audiences for live television and online psychic shows to this end, and many people visit mediums, believe in angels or have spirit guides.

Children often acknowledge spirit forms or ghosts (some believe they all naturally do this) in their play or in conversation with adults. Although they are not referring to what most grown-ups call a 'normal' (concrete, human) form, the child does not distinguish between them, and it may be a way of dealing with the death. Disbelieving, then, can be counterproductive. Taking these spirits seriously may aid expression and avoid unexplained fears or unresolved Ki causing tensions and unhelpful patterns in the future.

It is the effect these beliefs have on our clients that is important here. Do they find comfort or are they scared by them? Are they uneasy because of a perceived poltergeist, or relieved that the energy of their wife is present in the house instead of the emptiness they dreaded on getting back from the funeral?

Anthony C. Yu (1987, p.403) credits Confucius with the injunction, '"Respect the ghosts and spirits, but keep them at a distance" (Analects 6/20)' and adds, 'Whether this last statement implies a sincere presupposition of their existence or an oblique denial is tantalizingly ambiguous.' In Shiatsu terms, ghosts and spirits of the dead whom the living can see are manifestations of the client's Ki. Ki takes many forms and we can use our normal modes of diagnosis for these situations. From the point of view of the Shiatsu session, our personal view is less important: our aim is to respect the client, to listen and to honour their experience. Depending on our approach, we will either treat what they bring to us, or tune into their Ki as it is in the moment and take it from there. Whatever they have seen or felt, it is part of their presenting picture. We do, however, reserve the right to refer the client to another practitioner if we are uncomfortable (referral is covered in Chapter 5).

The practitioner who gives a session to the relative of someone who has died violently and feels haunted will want to support them during the treatment. Visualization and the sending of loving kindness to ensure the spirit has safe passage to a peaceful place are two techniques which can be used alongside touch.

There are those who believe in ghosts, past lives and other psychic phenomena, and those who do not or have not thought about it until something happens which changes their mind or challenges their former beliefs. Some of our clients will believe that they have lived before in a previous life or body, and this may or may not be relevant to the Shiatsu session you are giving them.

It is useful for us, as practitioners, to know where we stand on these matters, so that when our clients come to us with such information we have engaged with the topic and know something about it. There is a great deal of literature on the subject, and practising psychics or mediums are usually very happy to share their ideas or offer you a session. Sometimes clients will be looking for reassurance by telling us what they think or believe, and the individual practitioner must decide if that is possible and how to word a reply.

I was staying in CM's newly acquired house. He had told me about his grandmother who owned it previously, how she was a Reiki practitioner and spiritual healer before she died. He chose to have Shiatsu in the room where she used to practise. The minute I knelt beside him and closed my eyes in preparation, she spoke to me. Her voice was as clear as if she was in the room: she told me she was there, that she loved him and that she wanted to help. I held a silent dialogue with her, and off we went. It was a very tricky session and I was glad to have her spirit with me. At the end, I stood up to go and wash my hands and there she was! He had placed a photo of her, with her kind, smiling eyes, on the massage table behind me without my knowing, and it must have helped her 'come down', I think. I could not have done anything else but acknowledge her, because she was as real as the client was.

Angels, especially guardian angels (to protect and guide, help with avoiding spiritual dangers and achieve salvation), are to be found in all the world's main religions: Protestantism, Catholicism, Judaism and Islam. Vedic Hindus refer to *devas*, a Sanskrit word meaning radiant or shining. They are supernatural, sometimes referred to as gods, but are within the *cycle of suffering* to which all humans belong and from which everyone is seeking liberation. They help to regulate the cosmos against demons.

MW, a masseur, walked into my room as if there were sharp nails on the ground. She told me that she believed that someone was using their powers, distantly, to harm her, to try to kill her. She did not know who, although she could make a few guesses, and it was disturbing her ability to live her normal life (clinically this would be called a *delusion*). She had become increasingly nervous about going home, turning on the computer, or waking up in the morning in case she had a new, additional symptom or sensation or was going to die. I could not know if this was true, but her fear was real and I could work with that. Sitting beside her, my Ki felt scattered. She reported back pain, repeated headaches and nightmares, and her hand gestures were twitchy. When I did a body scan the Ki was uneven, and on touch her back depleted. The three elements featuring seemed to be Fire, Wood and Earth, and the Hara diagnosis told me Gallbladder Jitsu, Heart Governor Kyo. I alternated rotations to smooth the Ki, and calm palming on the outsides of her legs in side position. After ten minutes her breathing began to lengthen, and when I turned her over, she gave a yawn. She started to tell me about her caravan in the countryside where she felt safe. She suggested she could go there for a spell to relax, get away from the city, where she might feel stronger to combat what was happening.

In our diagnosis, there might be a variety of factors present when the client is reporting a ghost, spirit or angel: an emotion may be uppermost (happiness, fear or anger); the underlying state of mind might be more important, a sense that they are finding a way to deal with loss which is helping them to stay alive; or it could be a newfound opening of the mind at the realization that there is more to their life than the mundane. A spiritual belief of whatever sort will fall broadly into the Fire element phase and, depending on the effect, may cause the client to feel her Heart Ki is balanced or unbalanced. If causing disturbance, these effects may affect one of the other Organs or meridians (see Chapter 2).

It is said that our community understanding and shared skill at the end of life has dwindled over time. The dying, their relatives and friends may know that death is near, but not acknowledge or reveal that fact – some avoid visiting their relatives at the end of life, as it is too painful to watch. Deaths can arrive abruptly, immediately, painstakingly slowly, or there can be a long warning, allowing preparations to be made. Sometimes there is openness and a gathering of the clan right up to the end; at others, the client is dying alone. Within the same family, the experience of death can be vastly different, or the familiarity of the process the second time around can offer some succour at a sad time.

Shiatsu has a part to play at every stage and for all involved. Occupying a truly unique role with its attention to all levels of being at the same time, it is both a highly relevant support and entirely necessary.

The Practitioner

Chapter 5 is for you, the practitioner. When we meet death, whether in our personal or professional lives, the effect it has on us will influence the way we give Shiatsu. Here we will examine how to be supported effectively to enable us to do this important work, and there is a practical section on preparing for our own death, so that our clients are cared for afterwards. If we have taken the time to think and debate about grief and loss in the same way that we have researched and talked about techniques and points, then when we receive the news that a long-standing client has been given a terminal diagnosis, we have a better chance of responding usefully.

Facing death
We cannot avoid it
In Chapter 3, I identified just how many people are facing death, and how loss is inherent in so many aspects of their lives. Our clients cannot avoid it completely, and so we as Shiatsu practitioners cannot either. If our Ki is moving, then we are alive. Life involves change, and with that comes loss. Further, some of us make a conscious choice to focus on end-of-life care. Perhaps we have met death in our own lives, found Shiatsu helpful and want to offer it to others, to help them. Maybe we are drawn to this work because we want to learn more about it for ourselves. Sometimes we do not know why, but we have attracted a new group of people who all come to us with these sorts of issues.

Our aim is to support clients intelligently and intuitively. With a clear mind, we want to be able to apply what we have learned in our years of practice, to diagnose and make choices about where and how to touch. At the same time, it is imperative that we stay congruent and honestly aware of our own feelings in order to identify and empathize. Let us be honest, death is a situation that many practitioners fear, and fear can challenge these aims. One must be brave to make a true Shiatsu connection in these sorts of circumstances, and to know how to deal with them in an informed way.

Death and loss are emotive subjects: we know that, because we witness people trying not to talk about it. Even when it is obvious, we see people ignoring it. We are human, and most of us would prefer to live rather than die, prefer to be happy rather than sad, so it is understandable. We prefer to 'look on the bright side' and get on with our lives. However, Shiatsu practitioners also like to touch and be touched; we know it helps with life, and when our hands are in contact with a client, listening open-heartedly, we hear and recognize the suffering which is in all of us and cannot be ignored. As we give Shiatsu, the Ki moves back and forth between us, existing in the shared energetic field, and so it is inevitable that we exchange those feelings.

When I am happy and relaxed, confident and feeling secure, I have a sense of warmth and gentle fullness in my chest. That feeling rests onto my diaphragm so that when I breathe deeply it connects with my Hara and I feel grounded. This state allows me to give considered and heartfelt Shiatsu. There seems to be enough time to do what is needed, both for the client and myself – there is no rush. If they tell me something shocking or distressing, I notice that I remain calm.

When I reach out too far to care for someone, when I worry or wish that I could take away their pain, I have the sense of my Ki leaving me and my centre. I cannot always tell where it has gone. There are times when my client is finding it hard to lie still because he is so uncomfortable and this is upsetting for me. That can shift my Ki upwards, from my Hara to my heart. It can even disperse further outwards, and then I am ungrounded, even scattered, and consequently less able to help. If I cast around for my Ki, I notice that some of it has transferred to the other. They might suddenly ask if I am okay, bringing me out of myself, or even unexpectedly show further distress, and this can leave me feeling vulnerable and unprotected.

If we want to work efficiently and effectively with our clients' physical symptoms, we take the time to find out about the aetiology and progression of disease, and the drugs which doctors use to address them. We study and take classes, research, and speak to others who have those illnesses, so that when we meet those issues in our clients we can engage with them with assurance and understanding. It is the same with facing death and being with those who are suffering loss and grief. To be able to serve our clients well, it is useful to take some time in advance to prepare and learn about these states of the bodymind, and what impact they and their side effects have. That way, when they arise, we are informed and able to be helpful.

If we work with clients who have experienced the same diseases that we have, our reactions are likely to be triggered: those situations will have a different impact on us than if we had no personal experience of that suffering. We know that it is a good idea to process our own reactions and acknowledge the complications which were caused by the illness, as it will help us to be open-minded and non-judgemental with our clients. As we have seen, all of us will have come across death and loss in some way, and lived through similar situations in our own lives, and unless we have taken the compassionate time to start to process it, hearing someone else's story risks sparking our own. We may then feel unable to cope or to give Shiatsu in the way we want to.

There are some times when this sensing of the human condition moves us to tears and that is normal; at other times, we can remain compassionate without also enduring the grief. Our job is surely to stay inside ourselves, to remain centred and in connection with the floor, just as we learned to 'stay in Hara' as beginners.

Because we do not know what happens to us when we die, we find succour in certain accounts. We lean towards explanations which feel right or offer relief from our fears. Ordinarily these matters are private and not something we talk about with others. Death is scary and we need to be soothed, so stories about life after death and where we go have always had a certain fascination and power. They keep us moving on from day to day, help us manage when we are struggling through difficult times. More than that, our favourite theories are closely related to our reason for staying alive, even if they are hazy or uncomplicated. However, when we face them squarely, we come to realize that we do not know definitively.

As Shiatsu practitioners, we can usefully take the opportunity to identify what we think, or sense, that life is about. If we are clear about that, we have a better chance of letting our clients have their own opinions. As for death, there are many approaches to the subject and every one of us has our own set of beliefs. For us to do the sort of work to which we aspire, it is key that we examine what they are too.

It is likely that once we have looked into this dense subject, we will not be able to say that anyone else's views are wrong. What we wish for our clients who are facing death is for them to become still and focused in a Shiatsu session so that they can hear what they believe and what is really happening inside them. The aspiration is that they can be with, and move through, the stages of grief or dying which serve them individually, unhindered by our hidden influence.

For many of us, death was a part of our early life. For some, it will have been an obvious part – a dying parent, living in a war zone, a serious illness or prolonged hospital stay. The way the adults around us responded to these incidents will have had an impact on the way we reacted then and perhaps now. If they were open about what was happening and acknowledged it, this would have been different from a situation in which they had difficulty speaking or expressing it. To some extent we will have learned how to deal with our experiences of death and grief from the way our role models dealt with theirs.

RF's granny died on or near her 18th birthday. Her father discovered his mother dead on the floor of her apartment and RF was at her father's home when he got back. He cried and she had never seen him cry before. She described the sound and said she could remember it viscerally in her abdomen, sobbing when she told me. The circumstances of the death were particularly unpleasant, but it was the responses of the 'adults' around her which complicated matters: there were things RF's granny was supposed to have done or not done, and her role in the family was the stuff of convoluted family histories.

It was important for RF to talk and know about how the others felt so she could understand why their reactions were so different from hers – they were her family, she was related to them by birth and blood. However, it was also dangerous, because what she heard was conveyed through the prism of those others' emotions and memories. Later she carried on the tradition and in turn passed them on to her own children, and now she was worried if she had thought carefully enough about what she told them. Their mother's version came from her own grief and sense of (in)justice, and her children had to continue relationships with those relatives who were still alive. 'What I am concerned about is, what will that do to their understanding of death and what causes death?' she told me.

It transpired that she learned something important: that she did not have to share other people's reactions, not even those of her own relatives, although it was interesting and important to understand them. She felt that she was the only one who was sad and so had kept her feelings quiet until she was able to voice them all these years later.

RF's perspective was different from that of her family, and ours will be distinct from our clients'. Should we remain in shock from a death in our personal life, we will almost certainly be unable to distinguish our clients' emotions from our own.

Many practitioners know, innately, that working with certain conditions or types of behaviour is too much or too hard. It could be a cancer which we are afraid of, an illness which triggers some deep reactions. We notice a resistance in offering sessions to certain clients, or we feel inadequate. It is vital that Shiatsu is not given unless we want to, but at the same time, it is useful to understand why this is the case. Otherwise, it is possible that a client with whom we have been working for some time reveals or develops an underlying trait or new health complication and we are face to face with it anyway, shocked or unprepared.

Although Shiatsu is essentially bodywork and we may prefer not to talk much with our clients, by law we must ask some simple questions: full name and contact details, their age at first treatment and relevant medical history, including who is their GP (UK) or family medicine practitioner (FP) (US), and the date of each treatment – it must all be written legibly. As responsible practitioners, we take a case history and we are interested in ascertaining a true and holistic picture of the client: physically, emotionally, mentally and spiritually. Our questions are designed to show interest in all aspects of their bodymind, and of course we do not simply speak with them but we listen to their tone of voice; watch and sense their gestures and body position; observe their facial colour, lines and blemishes; look at their nails and tongue; and smell and taste their Ki. If that client is facing death and loss in some way, even if they are not telling us or aware of it, that will quickly become apparent. Indeed, we could argue that if we do not allow that information to surface, or miss or block out the signs, we are not using the full gamut of our skills.

Working with clients who are facing death and loss in some way introduces another dimension to our work. It might be interesting to note what state of mind is useful in order to do it, and whether we believe that it demands a different level of fitness and flexibility, asking if we have the inner and outer tools to do it or whether we need further thought, support, training and information. As it is likely to involve more emotional work than we are perhaps used to, we might want to pay attention to our boundaries and self-care, the preparation, time between sessions, and afterwards. Spiritually, it may call our beliefs into question, suggesting that reflective practice is crucial. Alternatively, spending time with a colleague, privately, or in a psychotherapeutic setting, having a healthy supervision or co-counselling plan which will flag up the subject regularly in a confidential setting, will offer us the chance to rethink and reshape our beliefs if necessary.

Giving ourselves time to pay attention to death and how it impacts on us requires energy, time and space. It is helpful to ask where and when to do this in order to make it as easy as possible, and whether personal issues are to be addressed at the same time as professional ones – usually it is best to keep them separate but sometimes this is impossible. Once we have some idea about what death means, we will realize the extent of its reach. To allow for adjustment of ethical and religious approaches as we touch suffering and witness distress, we must address our support structures, and this is the subject of the next section.

Support

The more we work with people who are dying, or managing someone else's death, the more we will recognize the patterns of Ki. These are blueprints for the human condition – the cycle of happiness and grief, love, fear and anger. The meridians of our lives both form and are altered at the same time as we respond to external events. We are retracing and laying down maps, pathways which are converging and diverging through and in the bodymind, which were passed on to us from our ancestors and will be passed on to our descendants. Exchanges take place between us and our clients as we sense their body under our hands, perhaps recognizing their sadness, and maybe feeling tired afterwards. When we are alert and conscious of the process, we learn how to stay centred and whole, how to be moved but not distracted from ourselves, and how we can manage to keep doing this work as long as we want to.

There are times when we are less aware of what is happening to us during our work with death and loss; occasions when we may not see what is happening. Many of us have been taught to look the other way when we see death or distress, apparently to protect the other and ourselves. Indeed, that may be the subliminal message the client is sending out: 'Don't talk about it!' Without noticing it, we carry on as usual, ignoring the signs, until something attracts our attention. Although we work from Hara, keeping ourselves well grounded, with our eyes open, and being present in the room with the client, we often have our hearts engaged in this work, and bodyworkers' hearts may suddenly open wide at the appearance of death. We talk about *opening your heart to someone* or *having an open heart, being open hearted*. Again, it is our humanity coming through, and while many practitioners see this as a crucial part of their practice, it can result in an imbalance.

The key to remaining balanced is to be aware of all four levels. In the same way that putting all our weight into one leg while we are working will cause us to be physically unstable, so if our attention is only with the client's body, then the session will be one-sided, we will miss valuable signs. We know how to use the Hara, the ground, and the receiver's body to achieve physical balance, and if we can apply this to the mental, emotional and spiritual levels too through spinal alignment and an expanded attitude, and an open mind and personal awareness, we will be able to remain in touch with the whole field, receive and transmit support from Heaven and Earth, and stay objective in the process. We will be using our whole selves and connecting with the receiver's. What a balancing act it is! We want to remain open and compassionate, responsive and relaxed, but we also need to be grounded and centred on all four levels to be able to meet those who are facing death.

As practitioners, we know that we must pay attention. Our physical joint discomfort may be alerting us to a need for a change in pressure, our thoughts may be raising our awareness that a client is disengaged, and our feelings can give us useful information about an underlying cause. Moreover, we know that it is our duty to ourselves and to our clients to be on the alert for signs of our own distress, fatigue and lack of concentration, for all these are signals that something is not right. If I am unclear whether it is me, the practitioner, or a client feeling these things, I hold my proverbial finger to the wind to find out which way it is blowing. I breathe into Hara, I expand my attention to my hands and beyond, and out to my periphery. Back and forth I go, asking, 'Is it me or my client?' If it is me then I have work to do, but I know that the edges are no longer blurred between our emotional states.

All practitioners have differing responses to working with death and dying. Until we start, or perhaps until we reflect on the clients whom we have already seen in the light of this, it is hard to know what ours will be. Some of us manage it the same way we do all our work and so it will not have an impact on our schedule or plans, in which case we can see as many people as we usually do. For others, it will not be like that.

Those who work from home may find that they require extra time before and after a session or working day when working with those who are facing death. Alternatively, it may be sensible to keep the practical part a little shorter to allow for more time to talk at the beginning or end, and so as not to overwhelm the client. If you are paying for space and are either allowed 15 minutes between sessions or have to pay per hour, even if you are not being paid by the client all of that time, then you might choose to see those types of clients somewhere else so that you feel less pressured. Working in a private clinic is not the same as working in a hospice or hospital.

The impact of working with people who are in distress should not be underestimated. Emotionally, it is upsetting to be with those who are struggling to breathe or in such pain. In addition, if we are in a medical institution, all the other staff you come across in the same building are dealing with it too, many of them doing it every day and on long shifts. This type of job tends to attract certain people: those who are very big hearted and whose boundaries are being constantly breached because of the perceived demands of the patients and their families. In the same way that it is hard for a midwife to go home in the middle of a birth, so staff who are attending a death may stay on to hold that patient's hand or support their relatives. This of course detracts from their own down-time, and does not always leave enough of that to properly recover before returning and starting all over again. This is the sort of environment that we come into with our highly sensitized antennae, and we can find ourselves exhausted at the end of the day. Hard though it may be, especially when the medical staff are doing such long hours, a shorter day is recommended, with a proper break at lunchtime if possible.

Keep a record of your energy levels and responses, be honest with yourself about how ready you are to face your family afterwards, notice what you are wishing for when you hesitate a minute and look out of the window, or how many times you find your attention wandering. Ask yourself if the schedule you have made is practicable and manageable in the long term.

Using the scale of normal

There are many reasons why mindfulness is a useful tool with those who are distressed. From the time we start learning Shiatsu, we develop an alertness to the different states of the bodymind. We notice that it is always changing, and each time we recognize this, we add to the body of knowledge which informs it. One minute we feel positive and the next, negative; sometimes we react in one way and sometimes another; after time off we know we usually feel refreshed, so we are aware if we do not. The more mindful we are, the more we notice anything out of the ordinary, and then when something happens we have the chance to calibrate. When we give a session and keep alert to alterations from this scale of normalcy, if we suspend for a moment when we are mid-way through and observe ourselves, we will be able to identify whether or not we are enjoying and are engaged with the session.

It seems that Shiatsu practitioners do develop a scale of *normal to not normal* as a result of giving Shiatsu to others – the more clients a practitioner sees, the wider that scale becomes and it is usually only used in matters of safety ('This is different from normal so I am alerted'), or to a certain extent as the basis for beginning a diagnosis, though not always ('This client says she has encephalitis, I have worked with people who have had that before, and in the context of that group, this person's symptoms are serious').

Being affected by the work

Working with dying people, those who are suffering extremely or have very sad tales to tell, can have short- or long-term effects on the practitioner. Reputedly, health professionals can be one of two things: either thinking they are unwell all the time because they are surrounded by the ill and unhappy, or ignoring any signs of disease completely. These are two ends of the spectrum, but most of us are affected in some way because we are empathetic. This can play havoc with sleep and the way we look after our family and ourselves. When we notice that a client's story remains with us, perhaps waking at night and thinking about them, it is a sign that something must be addressed, to take the time to understand how it is affecting us and clear our Ki in such a way that we can maintain inner peace.

What can we do?

REST
REflect, have Supervision and get some Therapy
(And of course, by therapy I mean Shiatsu!)

RE is a reminder to reflect

Beginning to work in a new area of Shiatsu can raise some serious questions, ones we may not have thought about for a while, or ever before. When we are working alongside other health professionals, we may be called on to explain how Shiatsu works. That, and the seriousness of our clients' situations, could prompt us to question whether Shiatsu is effective. Things we have taken for granted may arise such as how we know what our clients are feeling, how we can tell them what will happen so that they can make an informed choice, and whether it is possible to know if what we have done has been helpful or if it has been the cause of a worsening. In a situation where the emotions and physical sensations are extreme, such as a session with someone with a life-threatening illness or cancer, or whose baby has died, for example, these questions can take on a special intensity, even an urgency. Doubts and questions may cause us to freeze or withdraw, preventing engagement with clients who could be benefited by our touch and presence. In the same way that our internal beliefs change our Ki and can therefore be felt by others, so too any disbelief will be evident. We may fear that it could even result in complaints or accusations against us.

In such a situation, reflection is indispensable. Taking the time to examine what we did and why, the results (for both the practitioner and the client), and how it felt afterwards, is vital. Without this we cannot assess our work objectively, keep valid records and make valuable contributions to research, we cannot stand up for ourselves in all arenas when diagnosis and advice are requested, or develop our ways of working. If we do not reflect, we may be storing up unnecessary or destructive problems for the future.

The time when we notice we are being affected by our clients is when we must be alert, asking ourselves how we feel about what we went through and what emotions are around. It is necessary to reflect on any physical symptoms that are related, examine our current thinking or spiritual response to what happened, and, using mindful self-learning, to ask ourselves how we feel about death in light of this. We can do a self-diagnosis to establish where and how is the Ki. Using the Hara, doing the Makko-ho stretches and seeing what's easy and what is not, taking pulses, or looking at the tongue – whatever is familiar is the best. There are other methods of self-reflection in Chapter 8, Practical Exercises.

S is for supervision

Where a broad caseload inevitably includes a percentage of clients who are grieving or engaged with death in life scenarios, we may be managing well, able to incorporate these aspects of loss into the types of sessions we are familiar with. If, however, we find ourselves dealing with unfamiliar situations that are outside our comfort zone, we could find that our confidence is dwindling and there are questions arising. This type of work can, if extreme, cause us to question our relationship with Shiatsu and ourselves. We could find ourselves wondering if what we are doing is worthwhile or of any use to the client. Then we will know that we need supervisory support.

There are times when a Shiatsu session goes wrong. Depending on the outcome we expected, someone might get worse, hate it, complain or even die. This is why reflection and conversations with colleagues and supervisors are necessary. It is these types of outcome which prompt us to look at why we do what we do, how we prepare ourselves and our clients (perhaps also their relatives), what relationship we have with them, and which words we use to explain the outcome.

Supervision is intended to cover a wide range of possibilities, so that you are appropriately supported in your professional practice. A supervisor will listen to you and encourage you to listen to yourself. She hopes that you will find your own solutions and reveal your own answers, rather than teach or advise you. The sessions may include subjects such as:

- Reviewing your work with clients.

- Reviewing your practice.

- Self-awareness and personal growth.

- The client–practitioner relationship.

- Learning and training.

- Practice management (working hours, cancellations and so on).

- Business development.

Supervision is not the same as having a tutorial or taking a workshop with someone where you practise and learn Shiatsu (see below). For practitioners working with clients who are dying or responding to the death of someone, supervision is particularly important for:

- looking at the parallels between your own experiences of death and those of the clients

- having space to react to their stories and what they trigger in you

- checking your self-support mechanisms

- examining your up-to-date beliefs about the meaning of death

- reviewing your procedures

- addressing any relationships with clients and co-workers.

Some kinds of supervision are:

- one-to-one

- group (often cheaper)

- peer

- work-based, for example when you volunteer for a charity and your line manager gives you supervision.

ONE-TO-ONE AND GROUP SUPERVISION

If one-to-one or setting up a group, you can either choose an experienced Shiatsu practitioner/teacher or another sort of practitioner (usually a counsellor or psychotherapist) who has supervision training. You are strongly advised to set up a regular session to support your practice.

'Regular' depends on the number of sessions you are doing. This is a paying service.

Here is a guideline. If you are seeing up to five people per week for full-length Shiatsu sessions: supervision once every two months; if you are seeing more than five people per week: monthly supervision.

Note that if you are doing seated Shiatsu sessions, even though they are shorter, you are still meeting different people and their Ki. Make sure you take this into account, particularly if you are seeing people in quick succession, as there is less time for you to re-centre before the next engagement.

Peer support

According to Shery Mead (n.d.), 'Intentional peer support is a process of experimentation and co-creation, and assumes we play off each other to create ever more interesting and complex ways of understanding, much like improvisation in music.'

Meeting your colleagues regularly for the express reason of dealing with the topics listed above under supervision is peer support. It can be meetings with Shiatsu or other practitioners in the field. The shared understanding is ideal, and as no one will have had exactly the same experience as anyone else, even if you are all working in the same hospital for example, then there will be plenty to learn from each other. If you build up a relationship with the same folk over time, then the opportunity to express your emotions and deeper misgivings will increase. The regularity of the meetings and engaging with the same personnel cannot be underestimated for this reason. Once again, working with death and loss raises many issues for the practitioner, and a safe environment to face them and increase self-understanding is fundamental.

Work-based supervision

Shiatsu practitioners often work for little or no money. We are kind and generous as a group, but it is healthy to receive something in return, and work-based supervision is one way we can be repaid for our contribution. If we are working in an institution (hospital, hospice, care centre, medical clinic and so on), there will be a wealth of experience around and they will either offer supervision as good practice or it can be negotiated as recompense.

The Shiatsu Society (UK) states:

It is good practice to have one-to-one supervision on a regular basis with an experienced practitioner or teacher. During supervision, you should have the opportunity to reflect on your practice and to get feedback from your supervisor... Mentoring is not to be seen as a replacement for supervision and both the Mentor and the Supervisor should maintain the confidentiality of the client. You may also get support from group supervision and in practice groups; in these situations, you must not identify the client. Supervision in Shiatsu refers to a practitioner seeking advice from another practitioner (preferably at least as experienced) to review their work with clients and sometimes also for professional and personal development. (Shiatsu Society n.d.)

Incidentally, it goes on to add, 'Your client should be made aware that you share client information with your supervisor or mentor for the purpose of improving and monitoring your work and that supervision remains within the bounds of strict confidence between you' (Shiatsu Society n.d.). This can be added to the contract or General Data Protection Regulation (GDPR) form which you ask your client to sign at the first session.

T *is for therapy*

If we give Shiatsu, it is a very good idea to receive Shiatsu. I know one practitioner who does not like receiving it, but all the other practitioners I know, do. I adore it! Whether from someone who is just beginning or an experienced practitioner, it puts me right back in my body, connects me with the art I practise, and I always learn something: a technique, an attitude, a reminder of things forgotten. And I feel better, into the bargain. It can sometimes be tricky to receive it regularly, and many of us have other forms of complementary therapy that we love and get relief from which are almost as good. In order to avoid burn-out and perhaps have to cease this type of work, try making a list right now of all the things that are beneficial about receiving Shiatsu, putting them in order with the best first, and then write down the date of the last session. If it was longer ago than a month, ask whether you want to make an appointment right now!

It is so important for us to remember how Shiatsu feels. When we are working with clients who are seriously unwell or dying, we are offering comfort, and attention at a very high level, so getting it back is vital. Other therapies are excellent, but there is something about getting what you give, in order to practise with a particular sort of quality. It reminds us about pressure, penetration and body weight, which do not come from other modalities. We become the client who feels at one with the floor, and we also recognize that Shiatsu can sometimes be intense and uncomfortable, which we do not always register if we give, give and give some more. We are prone to just flow on and assume that everything is hunky dory for our clients, when they might actually be struggling. It is good to be reminded of that.

Then there is the matter of outcomes and reactions: although our clients are not always aware that the responses they are having could be to do with the session they received the day, week or month before – and although it is notoriously hard to explain to them that that might be the case – nevertheless, it is useful for us to experience it for ourselves. I do not need to say how powerful Shiatsu is, suffice to point out that it can often highlight bad habits, causing us to reorganize areas of our life or change our behaviour, which could have far-reaching effects. Our work with clients who are long-time smokers, for example, can bring them face to face with exactly what is in Chapter 3 – that they are dicing with death – and that is a very hard thing to face. We will benefit ourselves as practitioners if we are reconnected with this. We will be reminded that what we do is not just about bad backs and stiff necks, but about what caused them in the first place, and those causes can sometimes run deep.

Other ways to reflect and obtain support
Mentoring

On its website, under *Personal and Professional Development: What is Mentoring?*, the University of Cambridge describes mentoring as 'a chain for "passing on" good practice'.

When we are faced with incurable and indomitable conditions, and especially if the client is bowed down by it all, it can become daunting. In this case, a conversation with a respected practitioner who works in a hospital setting or who is familiar with clients who have particular chronic symptoms could be just the thing. The outcome of a mentoring session is recognition that the knowledge is there and that it is confidence which is the key. Sharing with an inspiring someone boosts resources and very often leaves us with a sense of the way forward, with belief in ourselves.

Working with a mentor is ideal for those who are new to this type of work or feeling jaded. We can all have times when we need an alternative kind of support, and a Shiatsu practitioner whom you respect, or who has more experience in this field than you, can be invaluable. A mentor is disconnected from our immediate practice (that is, not a colleague or a teacher), willing to listen, give feedback and share her experience. There are no rules, so they can be made up by those involved. It is suitable to meet in person or in other ways (phone, online and so on), and it is useful to arrange this in advance. Agree at the start whether it is acceptable to make contact outside this arrangement in an emergency. Money does not usually change hands.

Co-counselling

Co-counselling is a highly effective tool for personal development. It is a recognized style of reciprocal support within your peer group which has a recommended structure to it. No one takes charge: everyone is equal, speaking about themselves and sharing the role of counsellor. While one person speaks, the others listen. To be able to participate in co-counselling, you must do the training; thereafter it is often in pairs and is free of charge to all participants.

Tutorials

Many of us were taught to use diagnostic methods or to follow routines, and these can serve us well in challenging situations. It can be very reassuring to do what we have been trained to do, trusting that this is why the client has chosen Shiatsu and us as well-trained practitioners. If we work with those who can lie down on the futon or table and try it, then we can give Shiatsu in this way and learn and develop gradually as we go along. In the context of death and loss, however, we are more likely to come across clients who are in a wheelchair, or barely able to move independently. They may be restricted to a hospital bed with wires and tubes, and we may have a very short time in which to make meaningful contact. Our familiar Shiatsu may be impossible, so how do we proceed? Working more intuitively, trusting our instinct, focusing more on the energetic connection and on following the client's Ki are all methods which can be used when we find ourselves unable to fall back on our tried and tested ways of working. It can be most effective if we can do it, and a very good way to develop ourselves and our confidence. Here, mindset is critical. We must believe in what we are doing, trust that it will yield the necessary results and bring about the desired reaction, meeting the client exactly where he needs to be met. This way allows us to practise wherever we are and with anyone (within the confines of safety), and in practising we have the opportunity to settle down into our own relationship with our art. Whichever method is chosen, we are talking about practical work here, and so it may be really useful to have a tutorial or take a workshop to consolidate your way of working or get new ideas.

Workshops – online or in person

So, we have seen that there are times when input is unnecessary: it could be a sign that we are not recognizing our own skills, it could be that simply getting on with the daily practice is the challenge, or that it is something else we are really looking for, such as contact with colleagues. There are also times when we have been working with clients for many months, and a spot of inspiration in an atmosphere conducive to creativity and morale-boosting would be just the ticket! In this case, an informative online course or video workshop offered by organizations such as New Energy Work (Andrews 2019) or Jing (Fairweather and Mari 2019) can be taken from home, which cover a broad range of subjects, including interviews with authors, energy work training and practice management. What is more, you will be likely to share such activities with practitioners from around the world and so build up support across geographical borders, and form networks.

Finding internal support

It is most likely that what we need is inside us and that we need to find a way to connect with it: time to reflect on death, loss and Shiatsu, what they mean to us personally. Meditation, going for a walk and taking some time for a break might seem like stopping work, but in our profession these things are all part of it. They are all ways to locate our internal resources. What we bring to our sessions and classes with clients and students who are facing death and loss is our Ki, and the brighter and shinier it is, the more vibrant our encounters will be.

What makes for shiny Ki? We could refer to Chinese Medicine, to the five tenets for a long and healthy life, as it all seems to be there:

- Breathing and fresh air.

- Rest and sleep.

- Good quality and sensible amounts of food and drink.

- Study.

- Exercise.

In a convent, nuns spend every day the same way (Sravasti Abbey n.d.) – spiritual practice, work (in the garden, office, kitchen or community), study, community gatherings, recreation and rest. This way of living aims for daily harmony, rather than intensive work with a two-week holiday in the summer. If our Ki gets dusty and murky, neither we nor our clients will feel vital. For many of us, Shiatsu is a way or a philosophy of life – keeping the Ki moving means we are alive – and the Tao encourages a regular rethinking of the way we look at things. Dr Daniel Keown (n.d.) says:

> I am a Taoist, and it is all about creating simplicity in the world. Get the simple things right, change our own lives and be a beacon for how we can live healthily…we should be living as therapists, the way society should be set up!

This might require an alternative approach: if we continue to think of work as the opposite of relaxation, something to escape from wherever possible, we are attaching a set of negative values to it which will affect our behaviour. If from a different perspective we squeeze in as many sessions as possible because we know how our clients need them, we could be forgetting that freeing the Ki up and letting it play sometimes is as beneficial as being of service. 'If we regulate our own spiritual life, these abilities become internalised, giving way to the development of advanced diagnostic abilities' (Johnson 2002, p.120).

It might be time to reframe our attitude, such that work is as valuable as rest, and vice versa. That way we may develop a healthier mindset, and then our state of mind when faced with suffering, our awareness of the Shiatsu we offer and the littler things like the number of hours we work will follow naturally. Indeed, if we agree that we may die tonight, and that accepting this can focus us on life's priorities, then a day entirely spent working so hard that we have no time for the beauty of a river or the hug of a child may feel imbalanced.

Being a Shiatsu practitioner has a range of responsibilities attached to it. The mindfulness towards our self-care, and the aim to live what we expound, expanding the principles of a Shiatsu session into the rest of our lives, comes into this category, for example. These are not just for our own benefit. If we are asked by a client, 'What can I do to help myself?' or 'Is there anything that will help me before I see you again?', we might ask them back, 'What do you know supports you?' Or perhaps we will make a recommendation. But there is more than that.

As we listen to our clients, we will notice that they make small throw-away comments such as 'I thought I would try doing what you do and be outside more', or 'I guess that diet of yours is what makes your eyes sparkly'. They are influenced by us and the things they know or assume about us. From our part, we might make a throw-away remark when we greet them, about just having returned from the Sangha, but these things are noticed by those we work with. They are all part of the session and our engagement with each other and are therefore worthy of as much mindful awareness as others.

Here is a beautiful excerpt from a student's self-development essay about using meditation for self-support.

> When I discovered meditation and began attending courses and reading books on the psychology of it, so began an internal revolution. I started to see what I was saying to myself about myself, something I had never even noticed or heard before, and yet these conversations in my head had ruled my thoughts and behaviours most of my life! … The integration of meditation in my life, be this sitting meditation yoga or Qi gong, has given me awareness of the types of running commentary in my mind about varying situations or people. This obviously varies greatly from day to day, but awareness through meditation gives me the insight to recognize unhelpful modes of thinking. To perhaps catch those thoughts a little quicker, before they become actions. Awareness through meditation helps me sort the flowers from the weeds…the nutritious from the toxic, enabling me to assimilate the skilful thoughts and let go of the rest, so I can aspire always to be the best version of myself. (Jenkins 2017)

Supporting ourselves with meditation

Meditation in Seiza, the traditional Japanese sitting position for *zazen* meditation (see Figure 5.1), supports us by slowing the mind and promoting self-understanding – perfect for integrating end-of-life client work, recovering one's equilibrium from working with those who are grieving, and generally boosting the Kidney Yin.

More than that, Thich Nhat Hanh (2002, p.5) writes about the benefit of meditation in matters of loss:

> If you know how to practise, when the time comes for the separation you will not suffer too much. Building up a sincere practice over time allows the meditator to identify the ultimate boundary between one human being and another and to connect with the ongoing flow of universal Ki, thereby promoting non-attachment.

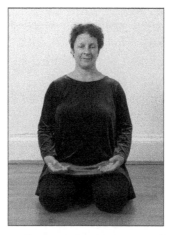

FIGURE 5.1: SEIZA, THE TRADITIONAL JAPANESE
SITTING POSITION FOR *ZAZEN* MEDITATION

Practical support for giving end-of-life Shiatsu

As we settle into this kind of work, we will sense that near death clients are moving away from the earthly realm, their Ki refining and preparing for the transition into the next. As a generalization, the more likely we are to be working on this spiritual level, the quicker we find ourselves moving down the meridian and around the body; it is less tiring for the receiver and engages his whole self. One way to address this level is with quantum techniques from Zen Shiatsu – peripheral awareness, spinal alignment, a light but deep touch (this is also covered in Chapters 2 and 7). The practitioner is contained and still, the energetic force is direct, and the whole bodymind is held and met at the same time. It can be tiring if the practitioner is not poised and relaxed, a state which requires fitness and focus.

Alternatively, many of our clients will be having Shiatsu for the first time and most will probably request some support on a physical level. Despite the assurances of certain authors, palliative care clients do have issues with pain and severe discomfort, even if not as a result of the primary reason for dying. As we know, medications cause side effects (in our terms Heat, Damp and Phlegm, for example), and they seem to require yet more medication. Shiatsu is really helpful in this area (inflammation, constipation, oedema). Maybe Shiatsu can cure cancer, maybe not, but we can certainly help manage these side effects or other, older symptoms which worsen or are still present in addition to the origin of the terminal diagnosis.

There is less sense of hurry when working in end-of-life care. The medication often slows the client down in all ways, plus the natural sleepiness and the deterioration of the organs means that life's fast pace is reducing, the client is increasingly *Yin*. Blending in and out of consciousness, taking time to speak or move, the client who has reached this stage is not rushing around, not any more. If you have held the hand of someone who is dying, you will know this.

Shiatsu touch might therefore consist of more palming than normal. Before physical touch is even made, the slow approach to the body, moving mindfully through the auras or light bodies as the hand descends, enables us to make contact with the less dense Ki where the origin or traces of physical symptoms are lingering. We may sense that we want to stay for longer and wait for the client's slowing Ki to catch up. What with the possible distractions of tubes and monitors, colostomy bags and sore bits, the practitioner may not have access to all of the surface area, and thus distal and off-body work can be appropriate.

Perhaps we find ourselves using a secure and positive holding position for end-of-life Shiatsu (see Figure 5.2), sliding a hand under the sacrum while the other is resting on or over the abdomen, or with a Mother hand on Hara while the other is above a wound or sore, and staying there for quite a while. This energetically connects these areas and allows space for the bodymind to recognize what it can do to bring about balance. Even sitting quietly beside your client with focus and intention can be a great relief for them, but we do not all normally hold positions for that long, as we have more of a tendency to keep moving around. Without adequate strengthening, this can therefore put a strain on the body and joints.

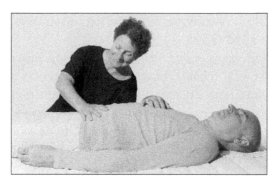

FIGURE 5.2: USING SLOW, LIGHT-HEARTED
HOLDING FOR END-OF-LIFE SHIATSU

We will have been introduced to various types of exercises when we trained to be Shiatsu practitioners – most likely the Makko-ho stretches, Do-In and some Qi gong. Sally Ibbotson (2019) explains that stretches and Do-In are not always suitable for those facing death. She says:

> It very much depends on the stage of dying and where people are – they can of course be active and able. I often use other forms such as Internal Qi gong or A Fragrant Buddha for both pain management and in the hospice. The latter has more imagery than movement because PICC lines (long, thin, hollow flexible tubes called catheters), colostomy bags, wheelchairs and so on are very much a part of the dying environment and practitioners need to have an adaptable and varied repertoire.

In addition, t'ai chi and yoga, as well as sports and walking, can liberate Ki and strengthen the legs and tummy. Standing Like a Tree, which teaches one to be still and rooted; held Warrior yoga poses for muscular control; and pilates for core strength are additional ways to support yourself in this kind of work, avoiding shaking and strain. Meditating for 30–40 minutes at a time trains the mind and body to focus and settle for sustained periods.

If you have been used to working on a futon on the ground, and then find yourself giving sessions on a massage table or chair of some sort (either because the client cannot manage or the rooms do not allow for a mat), this change can also cause added pressure, especially on the back. Adjusting the height of the bed is ideal, but if this is not possible then added exercises, as above, are recommended to offset the vagaries of bending over or holding a half squat for a long period of time.

Cat Westwood (2019), a practitioner from Norwich, says:

How to close the treatment is very important. I am a facilitator for the energy and person for that time and I don't want to leave with feelings or energy that isn't mine. This part felt different in the hospice: I would take 30 minutes after my afternoon, make a coffee, spend time in the quiet room that was also an open spiritual space, and I would take a moment to close before going home. I guess it was my way of having a healthy practice for myself as it was quite often the case that the patient wasn't there the next time.

Referrals, working with others and saying no
Why we might or might not refer

Working with death and loss is serious work, therefore there are times when we will be unable to do it or someone else can do it better than we can. The Hippocratic Oath states, 'I will not be ashamed to say "I know not," nor will I fail to call in my colleagues when the skills of another are needed for a patient's recovery' (Medicine Net Newsletter 2018). We, too, are bound by this statement. We strive to find a balance between fulfilling our training and our calling, and clients' requests, and at the same time recognizing our limitations.

There are some practitioners who believe they have a calling to do Shiatsu, an assignment to this task from a Higher Place, and that they have committed to that. Others believe that we have a duty to give freely according to our religious or spiritual beliefs, particularly in matters of life and death. If this is the case, we must each decide if we should give Shiatsu to people when they ask and do the best we can, or if we have a right to refuse. In these situations, we can call on a colleague or specialist to discuss it with or to fill the gap.

We may know that we have been trained to do something, or think that most other practitioners work with a certain condition so we should too, but in fact we have no desire to engage with them. For one practitioner, lung cancer is too reminiscent of their father's illness; for another, they may shy away from someone with a heart condition. For whatever reason, we reserve the right to say 'no' and refer the client to someone else.

At the first session with someone it is useful to ascertain their aim: for example, are they hoping to get better, get help with side effects or have a peaceful death? We might have to tell them immediately that we or Shiatsu can or cannot do what they request. We could discuss an appropriate timeframe for the Shiatsu, which is related to their medical treatment, or the time they have been given to live. And at this stage we may have to make a referral.

When we take a case history, paying attention to the new client's past health and asking them why they came, there may be a condition mentioned which we immediately recognize as beyond our capabilities. It may be that the client suffers from a disease we know nothing about (and do not have the time or inclination to look up), that they are really close to death and we are nervous about that, or that we are not experienced enough. We all have strengths and weaknesses and can acknowledge or name them, if for our and our client's benefit we feel that not only can we not help them, but someone else can.

It is good practice to review the situation with any client after an agreed period of time. It is at this stage that we can ask them how they think and feel things are going, and give them our feedback. If, before that time comes, we sense there is a problem or get stuck, we can follow our basic procedure (self-reflection, supervision or discussion with a colleague(s) or specialist agent) and, if it is clear that there is a good reason, instigate an early review. Other reasons for an earlier reassessment would be if the client starts to cancel appointments, misses planned sessions, feels she is stuck, or is getting nothing from them. After reconsidering, either a new plan is made and the sessions continue, or a referral may be suitable.

There may be sensible reasons why we cannot work with a client: recent surgery means they are still recovering a basic level of health; serious and repeated use of narcotics (class A) means we are unsure if they are able to make an informed decision to receive Shiatsu; mental instability means that we cannot be sure that the outcome will be safe for them. In such cases, we would be unwise to give a session and would want to ask the client to either wait (perhaps give them some dietary, exercise or lifestyle recommendations if they ask), or refer them to a specialist agency. There are times when the practitioner becomes unwell, moves away or dies. In these circumstances, a referral may be made to a fellow Shiatsu colleague, or, if the client decides to take this opportunity to try something new, to someone else.

Sometimes we must say 'no'

Saying 'no' to clients who are dying or grieving can be hard. We pick up their need – sadness or fear – and we want to help. However, it is also important to be able to protect ourselves. In truth, we will also be protecting the client. They need the best attention, and if we are half-hearted, depleted or otherwise unsure, our Ki will not be in the right place.

Referral due to the client's change of mind

It is true that we are human, we each have a heart which can feel broken and soft places inside us where we feel hurt, so it may be hard to acknowledge our shortcomings, our lack of knowledge, or a rejection. This is normal and needs attention – from ourselves (spending time alone, reflecting), others (colleagues and supervisor), or from the lay people who love us and can comfort and reassure us.

The decision of the client to turn down a treatment or to end a connection with the practitioner may happen for a variety of reasons: perhaps the client discovers what Shiatsu is and they know they do not want or cannot have it at the stage of their life when they are facing a life-threatening situation; it may be that when they are realistically informed at the beginning of an encounter, what sorts of reactions some clients have to Shiatsu, they choose not to receive it because they do not feel strong enough; perhaps they do not get a good feeling from or trust us given that they are close to death; or maybe they prefer something else. Whatever the reason, and we may not ever know what that was, we could be asked if we could recommend someone else.

To whom do we refer?

Many of us like to be part of a network of fellow practitioners and often reach beyond that to make contacts with professionals in other complementary fields as well as psychotherapists and those in mainstream medicine. In various ways, we share what we do with them, and they with us. We have enough of an understanding to be able to identify a match between one of the above and a client who is dying or requiring specialist grief counselling. When asked for a referral to someone who practises a different modality, for specialist disease management at the end of life for example, it is suggested that you refer them to someone you know and trust, or refer them to the national body who can help. Alternatively, direct them to their doctor.

If you are a member of a multi-disciplinary team in a medical establishment, you will probably be involved in patient meetings and/ or be part of a shared record-keeping system (for example, Crosscare[1] in Scotland). You can learn about the medical systems and hierarchy, and read who has done what and when with your clients outside the Shiatsu sessions, which will be useful. There will be medical staff you can refer to if it is outside your remit: for pharmaceutical pain relief, scans and x-rays, psychiatric medications and so on, and if there are other complementary and alternative medicine or Chinese Medicine practitioners working at the same place – massage, reflexology, Reiki – they might be suitable for the type of referral you are seeking.

In the complementary and alternative medicine/Chinese Medicine clinic or spa, you may know the others who work there, but you may come and go without much contact, unless you are leaving a practice room when they are entering, or perhaps making a cup of tea. On your clinic website, you can find out what they specialize in and there might be other opportunities to meet so that you can learn enough to be able to refer (such as at Christmas parties). Otherwise you will have to make an effort to make contact and discover their discipline. We are an individual bunch, we complementary therapists, and although we often hear each other say that we want more support through exchange, in fact we have busy lives and do not always attend and meet when we can.

How to refer

This is the process of making a referral if you are going to pass a client to someone else or share that client with another practitioner:

- Explain to the client that you are wanting to refer them and why.

- Ask them for their permission to share their records and/or have a conversation with the other practitioner.

- Tell them who you are referring them to, and reassure them that you will keep them informed of the outcome.

- Make it clear whether you are planning to or are offering to continue to work with them at the same time, or if you think it would be best for them to stop working with you and work with the other professional instead.

---

1   www.oneadvanced.com/solutions/crosscare

Developing a state of genuine humility allows us to sense when what we offer has ceased to benefit our client and intuit what might be useful to her. To conclude, building strong and informed relationships with other professionals or team members ensures that the client receives the very best care we can offer them, without feeding our ego.

Do not be tempted to act as a go-between with clients and their families regarding the end-of-life or other serious life-threatening situations. There may be some who are worried about leaving a legacy or have clear ideas about the funeral or memorial, but this is about leaving a will and related instructions and there are other professionals to whom you could refer them. They may confide in you, it may be moving, and you can encourage and work towards improved communication during Shiatsu sessions, but it is not the Shiatsu practitioner's job to carry messages or try to persuade someone to do anything. Use your supervision session to look at this if you find yourself doing it, wanting to, or feeling otherwise distressed about the topic.

Practicalities

Now, let us turn away from the grim reaper himself for a minute and regard practicalities instead. This section can be used by Shiatsu teachers who are giving practice management training to their students.

How to care for your clients after your death

By giving Shiatsu, you care for your clients now that you are alive, but how will you care for them after your death? Imagine you are a client of a beloved therapist who dies and think about the myriad feelings you will have. If it has happened to you already, think back to your response. The relationship which develops between a long-term client and her practitioner is deep and meaningful. Even if it has not progressed over a very long period of time, it could have been so valuable that both parties have a real appreciation, even love, for each other. Shiatsu touch can quickly create a profound contact, it is usually intimate, and much is exchanged within the session(s), on all levels, that is personal. The client will be on a journey of self-discovery, and the practitioner's role in her life can be pivotal to her sense of self – losing the practitioner will be significant. (Please note that the words *love* and *intimate* are used here within the confines, respect and professionalism of a client–therapist relationship.)

We all play roles for each other and it is not unusual for the Shiatsu practitioner to be mother, father, confidant and comforter. Perhaps you have been cast as adviser and healer, though you would not have aimed for that. You are not easily replaced and will be missed. Even the people whom you have not treated for a long while will be very sad about your death. They may have always felt that, should they need you, you will be there as you always have been, and so to understand that you are no longer alive will make a difference. At the least they may want to thank you for what you did. It is often the clients you have never reconnected with who, quite unexpectedly, have special memories of you.

The treatment room
TY told me that she had arranged for her clients to be able to visit her treatment room after she died if they so wished. What a lovely idea! Clients say that the treatment room is special to them, that they recall it when they are away and frequently need to reconnect with the feeling they have when they are there. It is clear that it is representative of something, an aid to coming back into themselves and relaxing, but it makes sense that they might want to visit after the practitioner dies. It would depend on the family being accepting of that and so a conversation would have to be had to that effect. To ensure that the room is left the way it usually was during treatments, directions could be left by the practitioner about setting it up.

Letter
Parents who know when they will die, leaving children who will be bereft without them, prepare a message or something else for them to read afterwards or when they are older. In the same way, you might want to write something to your clients in the event of an unexpected demise. It may be a message of thanks, or a wish for their future. It could be a general one for them all unless you wanted to write one for each, or for those who have been with you for a long duration.

Referral
It may also be worthwhile thinking of who you might pass your caseload to in the event of your death. If you are someone who has previously referred clients on when you have taken a break from practice to have

a baby, to travel or for another reason, you will already have someone/others in mind. Identifying a colleague, or more than one, who can both support your clients by offering them continued treatment and manage the effects of your death would be helpful to the person who is sorting out your business in such a situation, and to your clients themselves who may need continuous, seamless attention.

Legal preparations

In the summer of 2018, I attended two presentations by Kathryn Mannix (2017) of her book *With the End in Mind: Dying, Death and Wisdom in an Age of Denial*. Each time, she started by asking who in the audience had made a will, following up with asking about what plans we had made for our funeral. In our Shiatsu work this is not just a good idea, it is necessary. If I have a diary full of client bookings and a house full of client notes, by law I must keep them confidential for eight years (the Complementary and Natural Healthcare Council (CNHC, UK) stipulates eight years, the Shiatsu Society (SS, UK) seven), even after my death. If I die tonight, what arrangements have I made for that? A great many of us will not have made any!

Although the GDPR laws (NHS Health Research Authority and Medical Research Council 2019, p.39) state that 'any duty of confidence established prior to death does extend beyond death', there is no precedent set in case of this eventuality. It will be up to the family (if there is one), or otherwise the executor of the deceased Shiatsu practitioner, to deal with her *effects* (that is, every concrete thing and the electronic data, including social media, she has left behind), unless she has made other arrangements. Although GDPR is European Union (EU) legislation, it is enshrined in the UK Data Protection Law and so will still be applicable now that the UK has left the EU.

The Canadian Counselling and Psychotherapy Association (CCPA) advises its members, 'The right to confidentiality does not end with the death of the client and counsellors have a continuing responsibility to protect client confidentiality. A deceased client's right to confidentiality can be transferred to a legally appropriate personal representative of the client' (Sheppard n.d.). Furthermore, in its *Code of Professional Conduct and Ethics* (section 8), the SS (UK) states:

> You must make appropriate arrangements for the storage of client records in the event of your death. A member of the family within the

estate should retain them in case a claim is ever brought against the estate. If no-one is willing to do this, then a solicitor could be asked to hold them.

In its *Code of Conduct, Ethics and Performance* (2018, p.18), the CNHC writes:

> You are responsible for making sure that client records are kept safe when you finish practising or in case you were to die before this, unless you have entered into a contract that gives an organization or another healthcare professional this responsibility. If the responsibility is yours, it is recommended that:
>
> - you make provision in your will for the safe storage of clients' records. These can then be released to a client or their legal representative on production of the written authority of the client
>
> - when you close your practice, you publicise the arrangements that you have made to keep the records safe so that clients know how to obtain their records if they want you to.

So, who can you ask?

Someone who can make informed decisions would be ideal – another Shiatsu practitioner who knows you and understands the parameters of your practice, for example. Once you have identified someone, ask them if you can meet to discuss this and go through the duties involved, perhaps even offer to reciprocate if they have not already made arrangements.

Suggested checklist:

1. Identify someone or make a shortlist of possible candidates.

2. Contact them and set up a meeting.

3. Think through what you will say and why. Include the permission for you to share their contact details and the document itself with the relevant agent.

4. Following the meeting, decide who will be best for you and your clients.

5. Draw up a draft document, perhaps having a solicitor/lawyer look at it.

6. Contact your insurance company to check you have covered everything it requires.

7. Send the draft to the person you have chosen, for comment and approval.

8. Meet again to sign it – you might need a witness(es).

9. Make copies, one for each of you, and lodge a copy of the document with your family/solicitor alongside your will.

Keeping your records up to date

Remember to go through your records once a year and shred any which pertain to clients you last saw more than seven years ago (it is tricky because we never know when they might show up again, but if seven years have elapsed, it is best to be ruthless!). Make sure those which remain are divided into old and current and that they are in order so that anyone who has to deal with them after you die does not have a dreadful job. They must be locked up if they are on paper. Remember to put the spare key somewhere safe or give it to the person you have appointed – it is surprisingly hard to break into a filing cabinet!

Client's death

According to the CCPA:

> A deceased client's right to confidentiality can be transferred to a legally appropriate personal representative of the client. However, this person would not usually be a parent in the case of adult clients. This representative can then exercise informed consent on behalf of the client. Re. clients' representatives requesting information after they have died: We should require them to provide proof that they are legally the named person and are acting with consent. (Sheppard n.d.)

Shiatsu teachers – preparations for death

If you are a teacher and have a school with all the administrative and subject documents, or are an independent class/workshop leader owning files that you have spent many years developing, you will want to make provision for their safety or disposal as well. It is only the student records which must be dealt with by law, under the same GDPR rules as clients, but you might want your documents to be passed to another teacher or someone who could take over the school for you. You can follow the process as above for appointing a Shiatsu executor, although a fellow teacher may be more appropriate. You may have co-teachers, assistants and colleagues in the organization with whom you have agreed to jointly act in such a situation, which is a straightforward way of doing this.

Papers – accounts, insurance and so on

It is a matter of course that your family/executor will deal with your personal financial and legal affairs. You can choose, as you prepare for your death with a Shiatsu executor, whether to include the financial and legal affairs which relate to your practice/school/teaching, or not. If you decide in the affirmative, then these matters will be included in the agreement you draw up.

Remember, this is a big job for someone unless your papers are all in order and up to date. It is also a serious amount of work for you to do this for yourself, and not something you would want to start if you had just received a life-threatening diagnosis or were ill.

Somewhere, you will have to leave a list of usernames, passwords and PIN numbers for all your accounts, and social media if you use that, so that others can notify the relevant people. It is of course not usually recommended to share such information, but there will have to be a way for this particular eventuality.

Here is a checklist of things which someone will have to do for you regarding this aspect of your business (in no particular order):

- Contact your lawyer if you have one – this can probably be done through your family.

- Contact your Shiatsu insurance company (personal liability, public liability if you have it, personal accident (especially if it provides a lump sum on the event of your death)).

- Complete your accounts and those of your school if appropriate (they must be kept for eight years).

- Contact your Shiatsu society, CNHC or other professional body membership organizations.

- Contact your clinic, school premises and other relevant venues.

- Contact any organizations which you work for: adult education, hospitals and hospices, colleges and schools, including related subjects such as your Chi Gung classes.

- Cancel any subscriptions which you may have for Shiatsu-related journals.

- Prepare and file your final accounts at the end of the tax year(s) or liaise with your accountant, including National Insurance (UK); Federal Insurance Contributions Act tax (Wikipedia 2019) or Self Employed Contributions Act tax in the US; and Medicare levy (Australia).

- If you have a Shiatsu business bank account, email address and social media accounts (which is strongly advised as a way of keeping your private and personal lives separate), these will have to be closed and announcements might need to be made. Your relatives may not be able to get access to any funds which are in them unless you have given them permission before your death.

Other practicalities: appointments and cancellations

With home or private clinic clients who are dealing with death and loss, the frequency of cancellations or no-shows is higher. If they are very ill themselves, they may have had a relapse, be too unwell to come, or have a last-minute hospital appointment. If they are caring for someone who is dying, there may be an emergency or just too much to do to be able to leave them. If they are in the throes of grieving, they could be overwhelmed and unable to make the journey.

When you work in a hospice, cancellations are a feature of every day: even when you have said hello to staff at the beginning of the day and been given a list of who requires a session, your schedule can change within the hour. If you have booked clients in the previous week, you may find that they have died in the meantime, sometimes unexpectedly, been transferred to hospital or be otherwise engaged with medical staff, especially the consultant who takes precedence over everyone else. This is one reason why this type of work requires eternal patience and acceptance – it is a good lesson!

Fee or no fee

If you only have a few clients on your books at any one time, you could decide to let a missed appointment pass because of exceptional circumstances. However, if all your clients are in this type of situation, then you may need to find another way to recoup your room rental, babysitting fees and so on, otherwise you might be regularly losing out, financially and psychologically.

How do you feel when it happens?

You may or may not find out what happened to the client who did not come for their appointment. You may want to message them to find out, and, if you knew they were dying, you will be prepared and know to word it carefully. It may eventually be picked up by a relative or someone who is dealing with their affairs. Remember that it is possible that your client did not tell anyone about their sessions with you, so keep the message vague in case. For example, 'I hope everything is okay. Let me know how you are when you can' will be a prompt to a client who knows what you are referring to. If the person who picks it up does not know you, you have not given away any private information. If you send it and do not receive a reply, you will have to deal with the consequences, and your colleagues and supervisor will be there for you. This may be the start of your own grieving period – make sure you allow private time and have compassion for yourself.

If you did not know they were dying, if they had an accident or something else unexpected happened to cause the client's death, you may never know, or you may find out much later. In the meantime, your feelings may be complex. Feeling initially fed up, disappointed or angry in the absence of an explanation for a missed appointment would not be a surprising response, but if you then discover they have died, this could make your feelings more complex. Again, giving yourself adequate support will be valuable. Remember – there is no right or wrong way to feel.

It is very tempting to discuss such things with a partner or close friend, and although this is not legally allowed, many practitioners do it. Focusing on your own feelings and reactions is usually fine, but be careful about using names and private details, especially if the conversation takes place in public.

Clients
Boundaries and exchange

Sometimes we feel separate, that no one knows what we are thinking or feeling. We greet someone nonchalantly, but we are thinking how glad we are that they are still alive because the last time we saw them they looked close to death. Take care! If you ask them whether they know what you were really thinking, they will probably tell you. We hear the tone of someone's voice rise a semitone higher, even though they are saying 'Everything's fine', and if we stop for a moment, we can acknowledge that what they are saying and the way they are behaving do not correspond with their Ki.

We practitioners have spent money and time honing this sensitivity, that is our speciality. In fact, unless we remember to 'switch off' our antennae or 'turn down' our receptors, we will find ourselves hearing what folk are wondering, as in that film where the man bangs his head and can suddenly hear what women are thinking![2] This we must acknowledge. If we really believe in Ki (that we are all made of it as is the air and the floor), then it stands to reason that it is possible to 'know' what state of Ki someone is in – after all, we share, and all consist of, the same matter. If we are rushing madly to get the room ready, then the client will notice that our Ki is busy when she arrives.

On a good day we know this, we have trained ourselves to acknowledge it with the people around us. In an ideal world, we would give ourselves time to prepare calmly, but life is tricky sometimes, and so the next best thing is to say out loud: 'You might pick up that I am upset about something, and you would be right, but I am happy to see you today. Tell me how you are.' In doing that we are modelling congruence (aligning the way we are behaving with the way we are feeling), and honest communication. It is not simply the Shiatsu we give, it is the aura around us, and our mode of behaviour, which attracts our clients to us.

Giving Shiatsu to family and friends

When we say we are 'close' to someone it usually means that we share their Ki field or that when we are with them the edges between us are sufficiently porous so that more is exchanged across them than is usual with clients. Thus, we have a way into their suffering and an immediate

---

2   *What Women Want* (2000).

sense of their needs. It is more akin to our relationship with ourselves than our relationship with a client. This closeness may sometimes mean that we mimic the symptoms of that person, and may sometimes be playing a complementary role: for example, if they are in shock we may feel shocked too, or perhaps particularly clear minded and sharp; if they are in a Water state of mind and scared, we could be too, or alternatively, we could be bringing our Metal to the fore, behaving in an organized and precise way to help deal with the situation. Maintaining objectivity in these situations will be a challenge, and we are advised to think very carefully about the implications of giving them Shiatsu – how objective will it be and therefore how beneficial for them? How tiring and depleting, even frustrating, will it be for us?

In an emergency situation (a serious accident perhaps) when someone close to us is in trouble, it makes sense to use Shiatsu as best we can in the circumstances. The extent of our usefulness if we find ourselves accompanying a friend or family member to the hospital in the middle of the night will depend on our state of mind. If we are worried about them, it may not be useful to use Shiatsu or a similar intervention; in fact, a child most likely needs a hug and reassurance, or an elderly parent wants to have their hand held. However, if we find ourselves in a hospital emergency waiting room, we might remember that we have acupoints at our disposal: using Kidney 1 and Small Intestine 3 to bring someone round from an epileptic fit or faint, for example, or to resuscitate and keep someone alert so that if concussed they do not fall asleep, would be invaluable in such a situation.

Without thinking twice, we can switch away from our role as a friend or family member and morph into our Shiatsu persona, particularly if there is a second well, non-injured person present to perform other useful functions, and this could allow us to step into a more objective place and see the bigger picture, accessing our intuition. There may be things we can do to supplement the work of the hospital, ensuring that the patient gets the best of each approach, but it is probably worth asking permission or notifying a member of hospital staff before you do something, or otherwise standing back if they are managing it themselves.

What we must be careful of is not to lose sight of ourselves. Being aware of our own needs at the same time as attempting to give Shiatsu when we are very distressed about our child not being able to breathe, or our mother in severe hip pain from a fall, is quite a challenge. If we are feeling panicked or frightened, it is hard to keep our responsible

Shiatsu hat on. What is best for the relative, what role we play in this situation, whether remaining their family member or stepping into our Shiatsu practitioner shoes are decisions we might have to make on the spot. Being both practitioner and a shocked/bereaved person at the same time can be helpful because it might help us stay calm and perhaps identify the cause, but it can also add stress and even remove us from the familial relationship. Maybe choosing to relay their symptoms effectively to the medical staff in a way which will get them the care they need, instead of managing it ourselves, would be preferable for all concerned in these circumstances.

If a friend, especially a close one, is diagnosed with cancer or has a heart attack, we may well instinctively offer her Shiatsu. Wait! Is that the best way to support her? She is a friend, not a client, and the rules of engagement are very different in the two groups. In such situations, we are better off asking ourselves if we are sure we want to be bound by this, such that it is not easy to go round for a coffee without either being cast into the practitioner role or feeling we should be giving her a session when off duty, so to speak. Maybe we can find a way of discussing and debating things that might make her feel better, having an exchange without wearing our metaphorical Shiatsu outfit, thereby tipping the balance of our friendship. We have to be clear why we want to have this type of relationship with her and not a normal friendly one. It may be that we are scared for her and that it is easier to manage these feelings when we are a practitioner. That might signal that we could do with some support.

If the decision is made to go ahead and give the session(s), we must both make sure we are clear about money changing hands (or not) and if the time restraints and therefore cancellation fees are as per other clients; there is nothing worse than having to manage the situation caused by a friend not turning up in the middle of a busy clinic because she thought it was a loose and friendly arrangement. If the friend is in dire straits, realize that being moved to tears by her plight, as a friend would be, is not the way you would usually behave with a client, and therefore the basic premise has changed. Our codes of ethics are there for a reason – to protect ourselves and others – and overriding them can cause trouble.

Being a carer and a practitioner

If we find ourselves in the role of carer – perhaps a partner will not consider Shiatsu from someone else, or we want to look after a relative – we may find that we are giving Shiatsu both at home and away, or having to take a break from client work altogether. In the same way as we would encourage a client to have Shiatsu and a network of family and friends to support him, so too would that be good advice for us! As above, it is a totally different thing giving within the family. Clarity regarding when to give and when not, the balance of Shiatsu and other sorts of caring, and having time alone out of the house for walking, meditating or otherwise having fun is worth thinking about carefully and discussing with others and the person involved because full-time caring is exhausting. Remember, receiving Shiatsu helps!

The Shiatsu Society (UK)'s *Code of Conduct and Ethics* (n.d., section 7 viii) states:

> In the treatment of friends or relatives you should be sensitive to any issues that could arise due to any dual relationship as therapist and friend or relation. If you are unsure about this, it is recommended that you seek advice or supervision from an appropriate professional (such as a fellow, senior Shiatsu practitioner or teacher or a professional in a similar role).

What if the client gets worse or dies?

Now we come to a thorny question: What if a client dies? We might not have the chance, but if we address this before we decide to work with clients who have a life-threatening issue or who know they are dying it could be helpful. We will not know for sure until it happens as every incident is individual; however, it may be sensible to think about it anyway, given that – here I go again – death can come when we least expect it.

Almost as soon as we are out of our Shiatsu nappies, we have to face the fact that sometimes our clients get worse after a session, and this was discussed in Chapter 4 where a client went to hospital after a session and ended up getting better treatment for her lung cancer. Here, the topic is raising its head again in the context of the impact it has on the practitioner. We have engaged with this powerful work, we are facing our own fears and expectations about death so that we are congruent and our Ki is aligned; in short, we do the best we can. And what if the client does not improve or gets worse? What then?

The first time I came across this I had some serious self-reflection to do and was very grateful for my supervisor supporting me through it. (Please note that this example has already been used in Chapter 4). I was on the bus one day and a client I had seen a few times for short lunchtime sessions at a local business was standing next to me. Without any warning, she told me she had been off work because she had attempted suicide. Not only was I shocked to hear such personal and unexpected information in a public place, but I had not known she was in that state of mind when I last saw her.

In the aforementioned supervision, it turned out that I was happy to take some of the credit when my clients felt better or their symptoms improved. I energetically patted myself on my back – well done me, I seemed to have learned something after all! But when I stripped off the top layers of this complicated situation, what I found was a gift. Taking away three wrappers – the information she had given me; my initial reaction to it; and what I gleaned from my old notes about what Shiatsu I had given – I found a very brightly coloured, smaller parcel with a question on it: Where does the power lie in the Shiatsu relationship? We looked at many of my other case studies, what had happened and why, until I came up with two more big questions: Do I have any control over what happens to my client? And, do I know whether one outcome is good and another not? Underneath were all these queries about the role we play, our relationship to clients and to what we are doing.

The result of this enquiry was a revelation to me and it had a radical impact on my approach to my Shiatsu practice. There were times when I used my shoulder pain techniques and Tsubos and the client was better, but another time he was not. In certain sessions, my intention was clear and ineffectual, and in others, it was rather miraculous. Even taking into account whether I was having a good or a lousy day, I could neither predict the outcome nor bring it about in all eventualities. I had to conclude, after a great deal more consideration, that if I was unable to control the outcome, then neither could I be responsible for it.

That turned out to be a weight off my shoulders I had not known was there. To return to the subject of this book, in working with people who are so unwell, this is fundamental. If we approach our clients in the belief that we can make them better, and they do improve, we are something of a God; if they fail, we are who, Satan? When we put it like that it sounds rather obvious – you would think that I might have noticed before, after all I would have been a whole lot richer if that was my super power! I can no more save them from dying than I can save myself. I could relax. (Then I discovered that relaxation *is* powerful, but that is another story.)

Here is a folk tale about death, retold in my own words, the like of which is found all over the world. Storytelling is an age-old method of teaching us where the power lies in our lives!

A farmer was down on his luck. His wife was fed up with him complaining about the weather and the poor crops year after year, and, in the end, he was so sorry for himself that he left the village to find Death. He walked far away from home until he came to a beach where an old whiskered man was standing, ankle deep in the sea. The ancient turned and saw the young one and asked him what he was up to. 'I want to die,' he replied, 'there is nothing left for me to live for.' 'I can't help you,' replied the one with a beard, and so off went the farmer.

A little while later, however, when he had stopped to take a drink from the fountain, there was a tap on his shoulder and who should be there behind him, but the same old gentleman. 'I have been thinking,' said Death, 'why don't you go home and do something useful, for I will not be coming for you any time soon.' Relieved, the young man realized who this was and turned on his heel to do as he was told. As he started to walk away, he became curious and stopped, asking, 'Can you tell me when I will die?' 'In a week,' he was told, 'in a week you will become rich, and exactly ten years after that you will die.' In the tradition of such tales, Death handed him a set of bow and arrows for no reason the man could understand and sent him on his way.

Seven days later, a bird flew overhead. The poor man was hungry from tramping far and wide, so despite having no skill in hitting a target, he fired and was rather surprised to see it plummeting to the ground. Unbelievably, a golden bird landed in front of his feet – he was rich! When a second squawked above him, he immediately tried again. This time he missed, but in the very place the tip of the arrow met the ground, a sumptuous villa appeared, all ready and full of servants to look after him. Well, he celebrated and forgot the old man and his prediction straightaway.

Nine years and nine months later he woke from a dream in which the old man had appeared as clear as day, and the rich farmer remembered everything. He ordered his servants to make a sealed casket and put three-and-a-half months' worth of victuals in it. He did question whether he really wanted to spend that long in such a tiny place, but he did not want to die now his life was so good, so into it he clambered, issuing the order to sink him to the bottom of the ocean and tie the rope to a tree until the time had passed and they could come and get him out.

Death was checking his list. There was the farmer's name, and off he went to look for him, but he couldn't find him anywhere on earth. After searching and searching, he went back to his favourite beach to cool his toes and work out what to do, and it was there he tripped over a taut rope half buried in the sand. He almost drowned in the shallows. 'Who could have left this?' he wondered. He pulled and pulled. Imagine his interest when up came the casket, and what a surprise he got when he knocked on it and out sprang the young man, somewhat stiff from his ordeal. You!

Down on his knees fell the creaking man, begging, 'Please spare me, you can have half my riches.' What an offer! Truly he hadn't learned much in that cramped, dark place. 'You knew what would happen,' said Death, 'you have had your time. You understand why, don't you?' Seeing the confused look, he explained, 'Your fate is the result of your actions, there's no escaping it.' With that he got on with the matter in hand.

You may or may not believe that is the way we meet our end! If we have no control over death, and that relieves us of the responsibility to keep our clients alive, what does Shiatsu do? And what is the role of the practitioner?

When I stripped back two further layers of my metaphorical birthday parcel – my desire to heal and my mistaken magical powers – what I discovered in the middle was very simple: I liked Shiatsu and so did some of my clients because they came back for more. But, was doing something I liked, which others also liked, enough in itself? In calm moments, yes it was, but I wondered how I would feel if I was called on to explain what I did and why. Privately it was all rather exciting and freeing, but I was now back to what happens if a client gets worse or dies.

I had been giving sessions as usual during this seismic change. As I experimented with this new mindset, privately acknowledging all of this, I could hear my clients more clearly. 'Why have you come today?' I asked. 'To feel balanced like I did after the last session,' she said. 'Is there a reason you are here?' I asked. 'To feel relaxed, that's all,' he said. They were not asking me to heal them from their illness or bring them back from the dead, they were asking me to do what Shiatsu does very well: engage the autonomic nervous system and give them time and space to take stock and see what was required, what, in fact, could be done about the state they were in. Adjusting my approach relieved a lot of tension and I focused more on what they wanted.

That is my story and it may not be everyone's. It did not stop me using what I had learned and practised because often it helped, but it did change my attitude, and this was the only way I could work with clients who might die at any moment.

Not knowing your client has died

RB came with a secondary lung tumour, so we knew she was not going to live for years. She accepted that, and I learned a lot from her about keeping on living. We had quite a few meetings and it appeared that her chest was far more open. Her shoulders looked more relaxed, sitting down lower on her back; her upper back had straightened out a little; and her breathing got deeper as the sessions progressed. To be honest, I thought that maybe the Shiatsu was helping her get well, but one day she did not come as planned. Understandably she was on my mind for a long time and I kept wondering if I would hear from her, but as the weeks went by, I accepted I would not. I sent a brief message, but did not want to break my bond of confidentiality with her, so it was not explicit. I had no message from anyone and did not know how, where or when exactly she died. I could not therefore go to her funeral. I was left to make sense of this and to find my way with my grief and the implications for me.

Attending the death of a client

What is it we are trying to achieve in the face of death or in the face of a person dying? Rose Fuhrmann, Shiatsu practitioner, writes: 'One needs to empty one's own mind of all personal conceptions of death. I very much experienced this need when I sat with my dying mother.'[3]

Shiatsu practitioner Sarah Jane Churcher writes:

I sat with a dying relative this year. I held him mostly, then smoothed along the Bladder meridian. He was so afraid and my hands naturally supported his essence of Water. When I touched his Bladder meridians/ his back, he said it felt good to be touched there. Afterwards, I touched his legs and I found an Earth touch arise. There was no agenda, no trying, no certain points or meridians; just deep, still presence; deep, slow, steady breathing beside him. When my hands moved of their own accord with his energy and movements, I sensed that he didn't want to leave this earth at all, but his body was failing fast. Each person, and each death, is different. My feeling is to work with one's own energy, to be rooted, steady and grounded, to hold the client in the space as it unfolds, in unknown ways… [It was such a] beautiful, raw experience that I was blown away for a week! Being with him at his death was an honour.

Children, other relatives and friends may want to see as much of the one who is dying as possible, and therefore they may be in the room or at the bedside if we are visiting the client in their own home to give Shiatsu towards the end of life. Children, especially, may be calmed by our presence, and are usually remarkably resilient. Depending on our own personal circumstances, having others present may cause additional emotions in us. In seeing their situation, we realize we could be in that situation one day too.

If we are asked to be at the death, depending on where the client is, there could be hospital staff, as well as family, friends and pets present. They will all need to be taken into account. Sometimes we will have been able to build up a relationship with the others beforehand, but at other times we may be unknown to them. Indeed, they may not have known that their loved one had been receiving Shiatsu. It is worth being aware that unless it is an assisted death, the dying process can take a long time.

There is the possibility that the relatives will not want to be present at the death, and rather than the dying client being alone, it is the Shiatsu practitioner who might be asked to be the companion. The

3   From a letter to Kate Man, reproduced in the Shiatsu Society helpsheet on death.

end-of-life, soul midwife, transition guide or death doula is someone who spends time with the dying person and her family. Like the role of a birth doula at the beginning of life, their job is to offer informed and experienced support up to, during and after the death. Such training would supplement Shiatsu skills, might enhance confidence, and serve as valuable continuing professional development and education (Fischer 2018).

It is a big task that the client or their relative is asking of us in this situation, and we will be doing a great service. It is not to be entered into lightly and there are a number of things to take into consideration before we decide what to answer:

- Where will the dying client be?

- Who will make the decision to call in help or transfer to hospital if we are at home alone with the client?

- Who else will be present and what is their opinion of us being there too?

- How will we cope with tiredness, a possible increase in their suffering, them telling us something unexpected and profound?

- How will we fit this in with family and existing clients, including time off afterwards for processing?

- What is expected of us, our role; what skills may we require?

- Are there religious or cultural differences to acknowledge to ourselves or them?

According to many accounts which have been written, nearly everyone regrets not speaking more frankly about death with their parents before they died.

Going to the funeral/wake/memorial service/scattering of ashes

It used to be that the *Code of Conduct and Ethics* of the Shiatsu Society (UK) implied that we were not to accept invitations from clients to social gatherings, invite them to ours, or meet their family members (nor other work-related connections to do with clients, particularly if we would benefit financially). This was to maintain professional boundaries – it was felt that getting involved in their private life was beyond the confines of the practitioner–client relationship. Now that has been removed, but it does state, 'It is your role as practitioner to keep the boundaries between you and the client clear and professional' (Shiatsu Society n.d.), and talks about not giving them reason to think that you are interested in them in any way other than as a practitioner to a client. The CNHC (2018, p.22) states, 'You must not ask for or accept any inducement, gift or hospitality which may affect, or be seen to affect, the way you treat or refer clients.' A client dying, then, raises the question of whether to attend the funeral, scattering of ashes or memorial celebration, if there is one. This must be your decision and might well be discussed with a colleague or supervisor.

Being present at the chapel or place where the funeral is happening, offering condolences and then leaving before any wake begins is usually seen as acceptable, but it would be worth considering what will be said if asked what the practitioner's relationship was to the deceased, and whether there is any possibility of breaking the confidence of the deceased and/or/therefore causing any distress to anyone. Being asked to speak at such an event would not be advisable unless the deceased also happened to be a friend or close family member.

It is likely that you bonded quite strongly with the client while you were treating them, and this may help you manage the feelings elicited by the client's symptoms worsening or by your loss if they die. Do not think that because your relationship was a professional one, or that you did not spend long with them, that you are not expected to grieve or entitled to feel loss. You touched and were perhaps 'touched' by that person. You engaged with him deeply. A Shiatsu hour is not the same as an ordinary hour, it is longer and more happens in it than in other circumstances.

Death threat

Our relationship with our clients is complex and there is the possibility that it may deteriorate or become toxic. A client might behave unexpectedly, or someone we work with may suddenly exhibit unusual and unwanted behaviour. Receiving a death threat to yourself and/or your family is a serious and unlawful activity and should be reported to the police. It is important that you do not keep quiet about it in case it escalates, and certainly that you do not try to manage the situation on your own. In such a situation, it is good practice to seek support from a teacher, colleague or supervisor, someone who will then be informed about what has happened and can vouch for you professionally. It can help us feel safer, and we might need help during the reporting process.

Privately, it will be useful to ask ourselves if our life does feel threatened or were the words used empty, yet still potentially dangerous? If yes, our aim is to find ways to face this without causing ourselves too much fear. We can reflect on the case with someone sensible and compassionate, to see what our part in it was – to ask whether we were too trusting, when, in reality, there were signs. Did we put up with previous behaviour which we thought was harmless or temporary? There will also be other questions to consider.

As a result of reporting this, we may be offered protection, or wish we were but are not. In these cases, we can review our safety procedures (enlist the help of the police (in this matter) and look at whether working from home is the right thing to do, if we are careful enough about travelling to and from another venue at certain times of the day, and if there are adequate alarms and entry systems in place). Finally, we might contact our professional association or society in case the client approaches another practitioner.

Giving Shiatsu to convicted criminals

When I was giving a workshop in London on death and loss, one participant said she worked in a prison hospital where some of the men had been convicted of crimes which she found disturbing. She had to suspend her judgement in order to give Shiatsu. When I gave short, seated sessions in the busy hall of a high security prison in Dumfries and Galloway, some of the men told me that although they missed their families, they were scared to go home for the weekend, back into the community where they had committed their crime, because they feared for their lives. Here is another client group who are constantly living with death and loss and who have specific needs. I was touched by their appreciation of the Shiatsu and my being there, and if I had been able to return regularly, I would have benefited from contact with others who work in these settings and also, of course, from ongoing supervision.

If someone dies on your mat

I have never heard about this, but there is the possibility, especially if we are working with people who have extreme issues or are at the end of life. First, pay attention to safety issues for you both: when you first meet a new client, take details of their doctor and the address and phone number if the client knows it. Have them close by. Equally important is the case history so that you know if they are suffering from any serious complaints. If they are, then ask what would they like you to do in the eventuality of such an emergency. Perhaps they want you to call an ambulance, a family member or friend, or do something yourself and then wait. Remember that if you do not feel comfortable with that, you have the right to refuse treatment, or to inform them that you would call an ambulance because you believe that would be the sensible thing to do. Know your emergency number – if you are in a foreign country or travelling, the phone number of the ambulance services will possibly be different from the one in your home country. Your Chinese Medicine diagnostic techniques are invaluable: the questioning, looking, listening, smelling, tasting and hearing are your way to check if the client is how he says he is, whether there is something he is hiding, or something underlying which he does not know about.

Do you have First Aid training? If you do, you will have quite a different peace of mind from someone who does not. You will have learned what to do in an emergency and will be able to put this into action right away. If you have done the training, but are unconfident, this will either be because you are due a refresher (obligatory every three years in the UK, unless it was only a half day in the first place, in which case you must renew after one year), or the course was insufficient.

If you do not have the training and are working in a place where others do, then you need to know their telephone extension or the receptionist's. If you do not and you are working alone at home, especially if you are in a rural area, you may want to consider taking some training to reassure yourself and set your client's mind at rest. Then, you can state it on your website and publicity materials. If you do not want to, why not? Examine your reasons and discuss them with a colleague or supervisor.

If it is a stroke or a heart attack, a diabetic episode or a fit, rather than death (though these could lead to that), you must start by making the client as safe as possible and then call an ambulance. If it is unexpected, but less serious, such as a panic attack which they have not had before, ask yourself if you feel confident to deal with it. You cannot prepare for every eventuality, but some are more likely than others. It has to be said that, in most cases, the person would already be unwell enough not to be able to attend the appointment in the first place, or you would be giving them Shiatsu in a hospital or hospice where there are other staff to deal with such emergencies. Make sure you know how to call them, and where the red button is to be found.

Shiatsu in the community

If we are at work or a community event and there is a life-threatening accident or someone suffers a stroke, we will be most useful if we have an up-to-date First Aid certificate, or if we can find someone else who does. Otherwise, we can use our instinct, finding an ideal position for the client, using First Aid Tsubos until the emergency team arrives.

Humanitarian and voluntary work
Volunteering

For various reasons, we often find ourselves offering our services free of charge. We see suffering around us, we care, we volunteer. Many of us are interested in working with groups of people who cannot or should not have to pay for our services: certain sectors of the community (older people who cannot afford much out of their pensions), certain symptom groups (those at the end of life), or folk in dire straits (postnatal depression, homeless people, refugees), all of whom fall potentially into the death and loss categories that this book is addressing. This type of work can be satisfying and fascinating, allowing the practitioner to expand her area of knowledge, meet dedicated people and give some precious Shiatsu where it is needed.

Finding work

In terms of finding opportunities to work in venues where you can give Shiatsu to those who are facing death and loss, these are many. Chapter 4 lists potential places and positions where you might be useful. Social media (Facebook, LinkedIn, Instagram) and local Shiatsu networking groups (practice groups, professional meet-ups, congresses) can be great sources of information about charitable and humanitarian opportunities.

Once you have identified the area in which you would like to work, you must find out who is the likeliest contact. Check the website (the vacancies or volunteer opportunity pages), do some research into where the company or organization is located, what it does, and who are its current workers and what are their professional backgrounds. A personal staff contact is most valuable, as is a face-to-face meeting if you can get it. Colleagues who are in the medical profession or work in a charity might be able to help, as could friends who work in the voluntary sector. Remember to clearly identify what you are offering and why, so that your letter or verbal introduction is succinct and professional. You may need back-up in the form of references, useful articles and research, together with information about similar projects you have been involved in and validation from others if you have it.

There are also a number of pitfalls inherent in such work and we have touched on most of them already – the toll it can take on the stability of the bodymind, the need for adequate support – and of course there is the financial aspect. Without accurate data, I would guess that in the UK around a third of us make our living through Shiatsu and the rest do it part time, either to supplement their income from other sources, or in addition to a full-time job. In Australia, 75 per cent of the practitioners who replied to a survey in autumn 2017 worked fewer than 20 hours per week (including paid client work and unpaid administration and business for the practice) (Strapps and Hunter 2017, p.7). This might actually mean that practitioners can afford to do voluntary work, seeing it as something that gives back to their community and provides them with valuable experience. However, while being generous, it may encourage the employer to rely on no-fee contracts rather than paid ones, which is not practical for the long term.

Volunteering with humanitarian projects

Richard Whiting (2019) worked at a refugee drop-in centre[4] in Lancaster. He says: 'It was a great experience for me. I learned a lot and made some lovely connections. After a while I found the voluntary work was stretching my boundaries and [as] I gave a lot [already], I called it a day and turned my focus homeward.'

---

4   Refugee Advocacy, Information and Support, Lancaster, UK: http://rais.org.uk

Francesca Jaggs (2019) speaks about the mighty challenge her work in Bosnia entailed:

> First of all, I think it is important for practitioners to expect the unexpected. That applies to any client, but especially those who have been through intense experiences like war. For example, I worked with a woman who had witnessed and experienced rape as a child during the 1991–1995 conflict. It was like she lost all her boundaries. I believe it is not important which meridians I worked on, but my attitude. I felt a moment of overwhelm as I met her. Having been briefed by the translator about what she had gone through, I was not expecting this wonderfully open, bubbly, sexy and beautiful young woman. I wondered if this might be a 'cover' but then quickly reminded myself of the need to not make any assumptions and just tune in and do what feels right…ignoring my mind: no should/ought/theory.

Limitations

Here, we are working with clients who have endured multiple trauma – persecution and personal attack – and, therefore, have multiple needs. The complicated web of grief, fear and proximity to death requires practitioners to recognize both their limitations and their power. Jaggs (2019) again:

> It was 15 years after the war had ended (2010) and I spent two weeks in Bosnia, mostly in Sarajevo doing Shiatsu as part of the organization Healing Hands Network.[5] A young man came with his mother to our small outreach centre in a remote village. He was very quiet and the translator didn't explain anything to me, but he looked stiff and frightened. I asked the translator to tell him that the work was gentle and if he needed to say anything or didn't like it he could let me know. I put myself into a 'no mind' state, relaxed myself as best I could and laid my hand progressively on to him, that is, approaching through the etheric field with focus and asking myself what speed felt okay. Afterwards, I remember feeling glad he had managed to achieve some relaxation, only for a conversation to take place over tea with his mother before they left, which I did not understand, that seemed to get him back to square one. Even more distressing to me was that the translator

---

5   Healing Hands Network: www.healinghandsnetwork.org.uk

later told me what happened. I don't know the exact details, but when he was a young teenager, he had witnessed his mother being raped, perhaps leaving guilt at not having been able to protect her. As Shiatsu practitioners in such situations, we don't have the resources to get to the root of problems. I even felt quite angry with the mother, feeling that, somehow, she was partly to blame for her son's continuing poor mental state, but we can never know what is best or the whole story. To prevent giving ourselves trauma we must remind ourselves that we can only help give some relief. The people we worked with seemed very grateful.

How to support ourselves in this type of work and the benefits of it

Jaggs (2019) continues:

> We would get together in the evenings and debrief. The organization wouldn't let anyone do more than two weeks consecutively as they wanted to protect us from burn-out. All this is important when working with client after client with different traumas and/or injuries. For myself, I felt taken to the 'edge' enough to reach a softness and openness of my heart I had not felt before, but not fall into a pit of despair.

It seems that the practitioner's state of mind is at least as important as her technique. Both these practitioners are experienced, and it is clear that they offered great comfort and care as well as exhibiting self-awareness, which allowed them to learn and benefit from the situations which they were in.

Practising Shiatsu while facing death

If you are facing your own imminent death, your continuing work as a Shiatsu practitioner will depend on your health and what you want to do with the time you have available. If you want to continue, and are able, you may choose to tell colleagues and clients. It is likely that there may come a time when informing them will become more of an imperative – perhaps you will need more support from your colleagues if you get weaker or if you are making plans for what happens to your clients and their records when you die.

You may find that you prefer to do certain techniques and bodywork, but not others if they are too tiring or demanding; perhaps you would like to cut your client list so that you work less. Both of these scenarios may have implications – either you will see clients fewer times or choose to work with some people and not others.

Working when we have been bereaved

Bereavement is the act and period of grieving resulting from someone dying, and depending on who has died, there are different depths to it. Grieving for a child, spouse or partner, parent, best friend, pet or others will affect everyone differently, and you might not know in advance how each will affect you. You may give up Shiatsu for a while, or know someone who stopped completely in such a situation, or changed focus. For example, you may not be able to work with babies any more if the one who died was an infant; or you may have such an empathy for grieving parents after some time has elapsed that you make it your focus and volunteer for a charity which cares for that group of mourners.

One Monday I came to work as usual, not knowing that my friend who lived upstairs had died over the weekend. I was only just through the door, half an hour before my first client was due, when I heard the news from her husband. Her mother and the girls were there too, so I was right in the middle of their grieving and loss. I was shocked.

I spent a little time with them offering my condolences when the bell sounded and it was my client. I had no alternative but to explain to her what the situation was and she left. That had never happened before, I had never had to turn away a client at the door and that added to my emotional state.

I then had an hour and 15 minutes before the next person was due, and by the time I had recovered enough to try and get hold of him, it was too late and he had left, although I did manage to cancel the others for that day. So, I prepared myself and gave one Shiatsu. I remember that I acknowledged the state I was in to myself, and gave myself permission to do the best I could in the circumstances. It was fine. I hoped that being conscious of it and as aware as I could would limit any possible effect on my client.

As with any workplace, the Shiatsu room or clinic may not be somewhere you want to be after a death in the family. Spending time alone or with those close to you, managing the practical arrangements such as the funeral or other memorial if that is your task, looking after others who have been affected – these are all tasks that may take up the time and energy which might otherwise have gone towards your Shiatsu business and clients. For your own health and therefore the wellbeing of those close to you, Shiatsu touch may be a reassuring way of connecting and healing within a closer circle.

If you are able, cancellations carried out by you are ideal, using the mode of communication you generally use with your clients. You may have someone already on call to see those of your clients who need a session soon, or be able to identify someone soon to refer them to. They will understand, particularly those who have also been bereaved. You do not need to explain what happened or how you feel. If this is too much for you, appoint someone who is not as affected by the bereavement to make the cancellations for you.

Not being able to see your clients or visit the places you work to give Shiatsu may add to your emotional load, but neither guilt nor worry will do anyone any good. Be honest with yourself if you need help and visit a counsellor or supervisor depending on the focus of your feelings. It will not be the case that you have let them down, but in the chaos which is grief, it may arise. Do not take phone calls from clients until you are sure that you are ready to speak to people who are not close family and friends. This is where having a separate phone number and email address is so valuable. Leave them for later, or have someone else answer for you.

Your approach to your Shiatsu will be likely to change, and it may be useful to take the opportunity to work with a fellow practitioner or your supervisor as you move along this path. If you find that your personal priorities have changed, then this may affect your Shiatsu ones, and therefore any recommendations that you may make. Perhaps as your Ki changes your mental ability to focus and concentrate, emotionally you may feel unstable or highly sensitive. It may be interesting to write about this.

In my father's final days, I accompanied my mother to the hospice. At the end, he was only 5 stone (32 kilos) in weight. Instead of his psoriasis improving, it seemed to have got worse – his loose, dry, empty skin was all red on the sharp edge of his tibia bones. I watched my mum massage him with such tenderness. For a while afterwards, all I could remember were those scenes at the hospice, but they did make way for earlier memories of him all filled out again and smiling at the corner of his lip. I haven't forgotten them all, but they are balanced with others now.

This experience changed me and affected my client work and my attitude to life. Once touched by deep grief and loss, we become different people.

When I was grieving, I had to:

- acknowledge that I was

- spend time alone, remembering

- work out if I had enough energy to focus on a client as well as look after myself and my family

- spend time before the session, tuning in to how I was; acknowledge that I was sad and that it was hard for me to stop thinking about the person who had died; and consciously decide that, for the next hour, I would set enough of my feelings aside so that my client had my attention and care

- reassess each time if I was too distracted

- cancel an appointment if necessary.

If I cried while I was with the client, I realized that they did not usually see, although I know my Ki will have changed at those times. Often, I felt better for doing something which took my attention away from the sadness. In addition, the sessions were helpful for me in other ways: the client would say, or the session would raise, something which helped me understand what I was going through or how to support myself better. And sometimes I heard myself make a recommendation which I realized was as much for myself as for them.

Death of a colleague

Most of us work alone a great deal, connecting at the occasional congress or in the corridor of the hospice or clinic where we work. We love to receive Shiatsu from each other and swap stories about workshops we have attended and ideas we have for promoting our work. Thus, when a beloved colleague dies, we are bereft. We do not have many people around us to 'speak Shiatsu' with, and therefore that person was precious. We will undoubtedly have learned from them and shared a lot, so it will be understandable that there is a gap in our lives and we think about them a lot.

Perhaps a ritual, alone or with others who knew them, would be a fitting way to mark the event and wish their spirit well. Maybe, if they were known in the community, there will be a memorial occasion and that will be a good chance to tell stories or share good memories, register and celebrate their life.

If you worked together it may be that you have lost a co-teacher or that there is a room or time periods free that will need to be filled. Perhaps you are your colleague's Shiatsu executor and will have your work cut out contacting his clients and dealing with practical matters. Be compassionate to yourself and do not think, just because you are a practitioner, that this will be any easier for you than for anyone else.

Take time to be alone, and remember to cry and feel the missing of them. If you find that you are doing those things while seeing clients, you might need to take a short break or arrange for some sessions (Shiatsu or psychotherapy, perhaps specifically for bereavement) to support yourself. If this is the first time you have experienced such a loss, or if the last time someone died you found it hard to grieve, this time it may have a particularly strong effect on you, so be kind to yourself and it will seem a little easier. Taking the rest you need will allow you to move forwards with a greater self-knowledge and awareness when it is right.

Afterwards

In order to heal after the death of another, so that you can find love again, and keep on giving Shiatsu, it is important that you look it in the face. Spend quiet time thinking about those who have died, talk about them, examine your relationship to them before, during and now, get support if you need it, and allow it to stay with you. Be rigorous! If you notice yourself avoiding or skating around the subject, ask yourself if writing, singing or speaking about it will help, devise a ritual that might bind the wound, honour the memory and, above all, be compassionate with yourself.

— Chapter 6 —

The Client–Practitioner Relationship

While remaining with the subject of death and loss, this chapter is going to focus on the relationship between the client and the practitioner. It looks at expectations, things which get in the way, negotiating the balance between the practitioner and the client, listening, loving, forgiving, thanking, and apologizing if necessary. Coming close to death, whether at the end of life or temporarily, reminds us of key connections and core values.

Expectations

The needs of the client when faced with death can be grave and extensive. They may feel battered from tests and the hospital environment. Some new clients are sceptical, some hopeful, and some have come because they are simply at a loss, not having found the type of reassurance or support they needed in the hospital. Managing their expectations is part of the session.

We, too, depending on how long we have been practising, in which settings, what we have read and heard from colleagues, and our own life experiences, may have low or high expectations of ourselves.

For some clients, feeling better for the duration of an hour is really valuable, even if it does not last. They get short-term relief, describing the sensation as 'a place out of time' or 'like I used to be before the cancer'. If the client then has a positive body memory, we know, by report, that they are more likely to be able to recall it in another setting.

'Feeling better for an hour' usually means relaxing and starting to trust the practitioner. There is less need for underlying issues to be addressed, but focusing on the breath, on being comfortable and on them feeling in control is very important.

The more experienced and focused you are and the better prepared and aligned you feel, the more effective your touch will be. You may want to help and have a short time to do it in, but be careful! Do not zap the client as this is likely to sap his energy and be counterproductive. Rest back in your spine, make solid contact with the ground, be light handed and light Ki-d until you know what effect you are having. Do not underestimate the power of soft lights, healing smells and peace and quiet before you even touch.

What obstructs effective understanding?

Whatever information you give out before you meet, bear in mind that the traumatized client takes in less information than the healthy one; that someone in extreme pain can be confused and find it hard to concentrate.

WR came for the first time with a new cancer diagnosis. She was distraught about her condition and prognosis. Having heard about Shiatsu from a friend, she did not know much about it, so I spent time with her explaining what would happen, including possible reactions and limitations. I made sure that I wrote down what I had said. I asked her if she had understood and she said 'yes', which I also noted. The first session was very gentle as she was so nervous, but she relaxed as it went on and it was short because she was weak and it had taken time to go through everything. The second session seemed to be fine; however, she cancelled the third, and when she came back she admitted that she had not had the results she expected from the Shiatsu. She told me that there had not been an immediate improvement and that she had felt tired afterwards – the very things I had said might happen. She spoke as if she had never heard them before and, though I said that I had told her, and even showed her my notes, the fact was that she was disappointed and did not return.

I was sorry about this, but it was a valuable learning experience for me. I realized that just because someone says they understand does not mean that they always do, and there are times when we cannot do anything about that. Suggesting that the client comes with someone who can remember and understand on their behalf, perhaps remind them when they get home, may be a good idea. You can also follow up with an email or message, something they will have to refer to the next day.

Does the client know?

DV had had a chronic illness for quite a long while when I first met him. He came across as a forthright and spirited person. In the third session, he reported a bad night after each of the previous two. He also said that he enjoyed them and wanted more. With an increasing loss of sensation in his left arm and limited awareness in his legs, he reported that Shiatsu helped him feel himself. My instinct was to work in a more energetic manner and observe the effect it had, try to find some silence so he could focus on his interior, but he was adamant he wanted physical, strong pressure and he talked all through it, despite little response from me. Unexpectedly, because he said he could not feel emotion, he also cried. I wondered if he was grieving his loss of control. Just before the next session, he let me know that he had decided to stop Shiatsu.

What did I take from this? That neither the practitioner nor the client know the right way forward on their own – it must be a joint plan. I did not follow my instinct and did do what he asked. Perhaps it was useful for him to have expressed what he did and hear himself say those things, despite the fact that he opted afterwards for something else; I will probably never know.

It is not always easy to find the balance: the practitioner has expertise about Shiatsu and acquired knowledge gleaned from clients over time; the client has specialized understanding about himself and an instinct as he is receiving the Shiatsu (as long as he is calm and internally focused). Working with people at the end of their lives, when they might have only recently been incapacitated and are still hoping that they are more resilient than they actually are, is a subtle art.

Giving my opinion

Why might the client ask for my opinion? Perhaps they think we know, perhaps they think that they do not, they may think that we know better than they do. Whatever the reason, they are expecting an answer and there are various ways we can respond. We can:

- expound Shiatsu theory

- give advice

- say what we would do if it was us

- ask him what he thinks

- pass on knowledge from others.

It can be scary to have this responsibility, and can result in us feeling that we must answer immediately. This, in turn, can make us feel empty of knowledge. Sometimes, we find the reply just flows as a result of the impressions we have gained from touching and listening to him and from sensing our Ki. It is certainly a good idea to put off any statement or suggestion until the end of the session, or even the next one.

It is not good practice to advise a client to forgo traditional medical treatment and rely on Shiatsu, and it is unlikely that many practitioners would do that. It is true that if we get sick ourselves, we may choose not to undergo certain procedures or take medications, and indeed our clients may choose the same, but this is one sort of advice we do not give. When asked for our opinion, we know that we are advised to speak only about what we do and why, and not about right and wrong, in order that clients make their own informed choices.

How useful is it to be given advice?

Most Shiatsu training includes a unit on giving recommendations: acupoints, exercises and dietary and lifestyle advice are the most popular. As a way of learning about ourselves and keeping fit, they are invaluable. Students who have attended introductory days often report that they like the Do-In they have been taught and find it very useful at home. In contrast, if we are with a client and wait before giving a recommendation, we often hear them tell us that they are already doing the very thing we would have suggested. They know what to do to improve their health or achieve their aims, and what they need is agreement. There are other times when someone does ask though, and at those times it can sound as if they cannot motivate themselves or doubt their instinct, so a simple suggestion can be valuable.

Better, not right

Death and loss situations are more than likely to be such times, and yet are also when practitioner sensitivity is vital: it is useful to be able to identify the difference between a handy recommendation, and unwanted and unhelpful cheering up. When we are overcome, in an emotional maelstrom, feeling lost or alone, being given advice is very rarely what we are looking for. The animated video on the Refuge in Grief website (Devine n.d.) clearly elucidates the research and resolves that acknowledgement is the key. Being with someone while they are in pain, really hearing them say that they are suffering, is more valuable than any amount of suggestions proffered. However much we try, we cannot stop them (feeling) the way they are, but we can be with them and quietly acknowledge that.

Reflecting on what we need in times of sorrow can help us in our work

Most of us have been trained to come up with plans for our sessions so that we know where to touch. We have a toolkit of Tsubos and techniques we can use in various situations. However, grief and end-of-life work can be different, and discovering what we ourselves need when we are sad or grieving, through self-reflection, listening to the people around us and conferring with colleagues, helps us to find alternative ways to be with them at these times.

The client's questions are usually rhetorical. 'How will I manage without him when he goes?' and 'How can I carry on?' are 'questions' which indicate their state of mind and do not need answers. If we repeat them back, they will sometimes elaborate, give their own answer. If not, we can sit quietly and focus on our breathing and contact with the ground by way of encouraging them to do the same. If there is still no answer to these impenetrables, then we can ask if they would like to lie down and we can begin some bodywork.

Developing inner strength and confidence

Clients who become well or increasingly healthy will often speak about their Shiatsu experiences or make a recommendation to others. Those who are very close to death or seriously ill will not be able to say if we were helpful or not; indeed, we may never know if we were. Our work is private, and the nature of end-of-life care is that we will be working in more of a vacuum than usual, and therefore it requires a special sort of confidence. We must rely on our own sense of what we have offered, being pleased to have given service without public acknowledgement. We need inner strength, so that even if we receive criticism for some reason, we know that there is no way of countering that with client testament, not in this specific area of work.

It also means that we have a special sort of responsibility to the client who might not be able to complain for a variety of reasons: their ability to do so may be impaired due to an emotional state; they may be mentally confused; high pain levels may mean that they have trouble identifying physical sensations, and so on. It is, therefore, our own sense of professionalism which guides us and instils trust in the family, friends and staff who might be around the dying client. Being insured, keeping good records and working with a supervisor are all vital in protecting us if any challenge is made to that.

Listening

Listening is an opening of the practitioner's ears and energetic field to the tone of voice, words and other indications being made. It is the energy that we direct towards the client that shows we are interested. We hear and process the sounds according to our theory and instinct, interpreting the weeping voice as indicative of the Metal element, or recognizing the courage inherent in the whisper of a client who dares to say, 'What if I die?'

While we give Shiatsu, we listen for the gurgles and sighs of the client's bodymind responding, and to the nuances and meaning between the lines of what they say. Although the client so often apologizes for his abdominal sounds (trying to explain them as breakfast being digested), the explanation that they are a sign of the Ki moving makes sense to us. Sometimes it starts when they first lie down, their system already relaxing in response to the atmosphere in the room, to what has been discussed or their own thoughts. And later, coming at certain junctures, we appreciate the same sort of auditory feedback and are grateful for the acknowledgement of a touch well made.

We listen for the incongruence in the client which alerts us to the various strands of complexity when it comes to matters of death and loss – how they say they want to do the right thing, but indicate that they are avoiding what that might entail for fear of having to watch their loved one suffer.

As practitioners, we also listen to ourselves when giving a session, listen to our own reactions. Thus, when the client says 'I managed well at the funeral' and I notice a sagging sensation in my solar plexus, I know to say back, 'And where in your body is "I managed well at the funeral"?' (a Clean Question). My bodymind is giving me valuable diagnostic information.

We also listen inside ourselves, for a word or a tune, a complaint or question, for example. In the quiet of a session, as I palmed down my client's back, I once heard the words of a Wendell Berry (2012) poem being spoken in my mind, 'I come into the peace of wild things who do not tax their lives with forethought of grief', and I assumed I had heard those words for a reason. I let them resonate in me, in connection with him. He cried silently.

I listen to the sounds inside myself, around me in the room, and even outside it: when one of my cranial bones adjusts or I bring up some wind, I know something might have shifted in the client. If I become aware of the clock ticking or if they start bell ringing in the church next door, I notice that, wondering if there is a reason and if the environmental Ki is telling me something (with time passing, the Water element – for whom the bell tolls, for example).

Then there is listening to the Ki. We talk about it a lot! When we use that phrase, we mean that we are open to information coming from the many aspects of the bodymind (physical, mental, spiritual, emotional, meridians, Tsubos, voice, appearance, gesture and so on). We mean that we do not have too much of an advance plan, but will respond to the messages which we perceive are coming from the client and ourselves; or that within the advance plan there will be room to respond to the feedback we get from the client and adjust accordingly.

That is where we attribute the main 'knowing': to the Ki. We trust the Ki and believe that if we listen to it, it will tell us what we need to know to make the session effective. The Ki takes precedence over the mind, the cognitive brain, although it is also part of it. It emanates from our core, carries inherited knowledge and feeds on the Universal Source. I thumb along the Heart (HT) meridian with one hand, the other on their Hara, and when I get to HT 3 something under that Mother hand attracts my attention and I listen to it. I might react in various ways: going deeper, staying longer, recognizing that it is an important point to return to later; and when I do, the client reacts by making a noise and I hear it. This is a chain reaction, established because I was listening to the Ki.

When working in the area of death and loss, listening is even more important than usual. Someone who is stretched to their limit, who is strung out with sorrow, or whose Ki is hidden inside a protective shell, might have less awareness of what they need or how it feels. When the practitioner listens deeply to the client's Ki, it can be heard. The very echo of humanity is what we hear when we work with the grieving and the scared. We hear the longing and the sadness, the desolation and the tiredness. It moves through us and connects with our own experiences. When I work with bereaved mothers, I sometimes recall a time when I dropped to my knees on the kitchen floor and wailed for myself, my mother and at the same time for all the other women who had lost their babies back through the ages. I am careful not to overlay my loss onto theirs, but a channel opened when that happened to me, allowing me to empathize.

When we listen with open hearts, the reverberations ricochet through us and we create a sounding board against which the echo can happen. The words can then bounce back off us, so that they can be heard by the client and understood better, they can then pity themselves, a healthy response. If I am grounded, I can help the excess to be disseminated into the air, for example with their arm in a Large Intestine meridian stretch as I exhale; or rooted into the earth, for example through lifting his legs, bending his knees, placing his soles flat on the mat and leaning back with my hands at the backs of his knees (thereby opening the hips and descending the Ki through the ST meridian). In the air and the earth, those feelings do no harm, they merge with the rest of mankind's woes.

You and your client are united through the suffering of the human condition which is at once wonderful and terrible. You will be left with a greater understanding of the client and of the 'bigger picture' (the 'What is the point of it all?' type of question for yourself), but you might also have suffered. Take care to sit with that, be understanding of yourself, allow time, or it will wake you up at night, spill into other areas of your life, or cause you suffering.

Finally, it is said that listening is what the Heart needs. The Shen, the Heart spirit, has to reside in the Heart for the Blood to rest, to achieve calm and relaxation. Although the Heart is likened to the Emperor, it has a slight and delicate Ki, with not a hint of the entitled about it. The Shen has a tendency to scatter, to stray away from a Heart which is coping with shock or danger, to look for a better, more settled place where someone will listen to its distress. Many of the scenarios listed in Chapter 3 will elicit that type of response. To remedy, a gentle but embodied palm over CV 17, maybe also a second one between the shoulder blades, together with a listening quality to your Ki – you can listen to the pulse, the Blood, the breathing, anything which relates to the Upper Burner – will attract the dispersed Shen back into the Heart to be heard.

Love

In the film *Collateral Beauty*, Edward Norton's character Whit says, 'I wasn't feeling love, I had become love' (Loeb 2016).

Love is at the root of Shiatsu. This incorporates kindness and generosity of spirit. The type of love the Shiatsu practitioner engages with in the therapeutic relationship is not sexual or familial, but of the universal kind. No special techniques happen in the session, it is still the simple laying on of hands, but to open, to listen, to connect and to accept are acts of love, and it is felt.

When Alice Whieldon (2018) spoke passionately in her workshop in Vienna, Austria, about the type of connection that must happen at the start of a Seiki session, it was about opening a channel through which love can flow. To begin a session with a grieving or imminently dying client by honestly settling into oneself, allowing a choice of where to touch, making that contact with respect, waiting for the awareness of the Ki between you to grow and be the reason for what happens next – that is both an act of, and creates the possibility for, love.

I do not set out to love, nor do I aim to be loving. Rather, it is a by-product of the things listed above which I do try to do. Of these things, honesty and integrity are the greatest. The Shiatsu practitioner is not trained to love, but the result of good practice (of meditation and energy work, of mindful reflection) is that it is there. To be open, to follow the Ki, to sit still with what arises – these things allow love to be there and can be interpreted as love.

It is being loved in this way which moves and brings about change in the client. It is intrinsically safe, in as much as the receiver does not have to concern themselves with the practitioner because he knows that love will be there, whatever happens. Then it allows the receiver to notice themselves, their Ki, and attend to what needs to be done. It creates relaxation which in turn expands the physical body in the same way that Shiatsu opens the airways or the blood vessels. That is what the deep exhalation that sometimes happens at the start, or the sound of the movement of something in the Hara, signifies. It acknowledges the presence of love.

In Shiatsu, our human existence is paramount, in the room and in the relationship. We do not spiritually absent ourselves from the treatment room, but instead we are present. We have our 'feet on the ground': we hear our own voice as we speak, sense our own gestures as we listen, and know where we are in space as we touch. It is our own state of love which we can feel.

What is felt by the receiver can be interpreted in their own way. They might describe it as God's love, it does not matter. It is the state which comes about as a result of feeling loved which brings about change. Sometimes the client will recognize and name it during the session, but often, especially in crisis situations (maybe a client who has been starving herself to death), it is something that enables them to feel helped. The focus is on the change, not the reason why that was made possible.

For the practitioner, love is our reward – to feel the love flowing satisfies a basic human need. We are grateful for the opportunity to love another. We may be paid for the session or not, but this love is often our reason for keeping on doing it. When the client's pain does not improve, if she gets worse or dies, love is one of the things that makes the difference.

Depending on our beliefs, the presence of love between the therapist and the client may be healing for things we have done in our past lives, our human duty, the reason for our existence, or a way to enlightenment.

Here are some typical practitioner questions that arise in the face of death. If the client dies, does that alter the experience of love that was felt in the final session? Did I love enough? Or too much? If the client gets worse, is it worth it? If they die, do I love for nothing? These are normal responses to extreme or unwanted situations. The answers depend on your beliefs, and your faith in love and Shiatsu. What is true is that it has already happened the way it did and cannot now be altered. You might question that love 'knows no bounds' if you are grieving for your client. Although it is not usually necessary to question love, you might find yourself closing up, not finding it easy to let the Ki flow, or even putting off doing Shiatsu again, and that is a sign that you need time to reflect.

Does death change the meaning of love in the Shiatsu context? If, after the session, you discover that the client got worse, then possibly. It will not change it for the client for whom you felt it, but you might, in your distress, feel differently about it. It depends on where you are in your Shiatsu practice and your life, whether it has happened before with someone, if you can accept it. In this context (that is, professional and respectfully boundaried love), it is usually acceptable. Luckily, once expressed, it cannot be taken back. Both the practitioner and client can withdraw from this type of relationship if necessary, and no harm will have been done.

Can we be sure the other has felt it? This is a matter of opinion, too. It can be argued that whatever one human feels, the other picks it up in some way. I believe that we do feel love when it is there – that is why we hear stories told about the encounter years after the event, and why clients often return a long time later when they are faced with a new difficulty. They remember that we cared, and they trust us.

Many elderly people at the end of their lives have been alone for a long time, after a spouse died or having outlived their children. Being loved may be something that does not happen to that client often, certainly not with a stranger. It is almost always something they did not expect if they have not had Shiatsu before. It could be a surprise (for example, I did not think I was loveable with this rash all over me; because I am weak; because I am reliant on others). It is not usually verbally asked for, but there may be a gestural request, or an underlying tone of voice that expresses the need.

Love is private and shared. Each knows that the other felt it and that is enough. It is therefore not often spoken about at the end of the session, though a heartfelt thanks, a pronounced eye-to-eye contact or a brief touch from them on goodbye probably refers to it. It might cause the client to cry, and you might cry too, because love can flow in both directions. As practitioners, we need to know how to deal with this, to speak about it, be listened to and believed. On account of client confidentiality, we do not discuss the specifics outside the session, not unless we are students or in supervision.

Feeling what they do

If love is present between you, then you can experience what they do (on all levels). It is my experience that the symptoms, thoughts or feelings that belong to the client pass through me, fleetingly, just long enough for me to identify them and/or make theoretical associations that might be of use in the session. Sometimes they are things I already know about the client and am happy to be reminded of, other times it is new information.

Any sensations or feelings left after the session should be noted and, when appropriate, addressed.

Shiatsu love can become addictive

This love bug could become addictive, or it might fill in a gap for the practitioner who is lonely or does not have the love around them which they need. This sort of connection is very powerful and it is usually recognized as such because of the universality of it. It does mean that one might inappropriately return to the therapeutic relationship to find it, so, once again, reflection and supervision are vital in order to examine one's motives and check that they are in line with good practice and one's ethical beliefs.

Bearing witness to others' suffering can be too much

Some students and graduates do not go on to practise Shiatsu, and some practitioners stop or retire, and loving and bearing witness to others' suffering is one reason why. They know that it is too much for them to bear (perhaps they do not have the support necessary), or that it depletes them, using up too much energy which is maybe needed in caring for family members or themselves instead.

One must be brave to make that connection with love, resilient to sustain it, and experienced in dealing with it. Our three-year training allows us to start to touch this depth of connection, in a way that a much shorter period of training does not. Although acupuncturists, homeopaths, psychotherapists and osteopaths all train for as long as we do (or longer), it is our very special combination of touch, words and range – not only physical and practical techniques but also emotional and spiritual therapy – together with reflection, that makes Shiatsu particular, and allows us to work highly effectively with serious conditions and in end-of-life care.

When love is not there, its absence leaves the client alone with their feelings (physical and emotional), the touch is perfunctory, the words automatic, the session practical. Love is the ingredient that turns a mechanical session into a transformative one.

Protecting our profession – love and rules

Even writing about this makes me nervous! We are just not encouraged to write about love and touch therapy in the same sentence. It is as if the possibility of it becoming abusive stops us from speaking about it, but on the contrary, what has to be said is that we must do Shiatsu for the right reasons. We cannot be 100 per cent sure that we would recognize someone who enters our profession for the purpose of gaining access to vulnerable people, or that we do not pass a student at the end of their training who might take advantage of a client, but there are safeguards in place. The extent of our care in training, our emphasis on honesty and self-awareness, the fact that we are face-to-face most of the time (as opposed to the people who offer undergraduate Shiatsu training online or by post), and that there must be three or more teachers over a period of three or more years, all of that is our way of rigorously regulating our profession.

Where there is a more likely gap, I would be so bold as to say, is with busy practitioners who refuse high-quality supervision or very part-time ones who do not engage in continuing professional development activities. Both supervision and continuing professional development are encouraged by our professional associations, but it is very interesting that we resist making supervision compulsory (in the UK) when every member of the medical profession and all properly qualified therapists must do it in order to practise. Upholding stringent rules is a matter for frequent complaint – the training is too long, continuing professional development is too expensive – but they are the way we signal to the world that we are responsible practitioners. If we want to work among consultants and doctors, at university level in educational institutions and with examining boards, and be taken seriously by researchers and policy makers, we must ensure that we are scrupulous in our prerequisites for practice. Then we can talk about love.

Other emotional reactions

Some people cry when their loved one dies and some do not. Crying is a response to a myriad of emotions, not only sadness, although sadness is usually part of it. If you want to know why they are doing it, ask, do not assume. Sometimes the tears are unspecific or of unknown origin.

We rarely cry if we think that the person we are with is disapproving or the situation we are in is dangerous. If the practitioner is not disturbed by the client crying, then the latter is free to do so if they like. There are some responses that we can make which give the impression that the client should stop, for example offering a tissue for them to dry their eyes. (Although, if they are clearly casting around looking for one, that is another matter and it is useful to have a box in the room for such eventualities.) If you are giving bodywork when it happens, stopping to ask them if they are okay is an interruption to you both. If you do want to engage in conversation, ask an open question (that is, one which carries no implication that you are guessing what the answer is or are expecting a certain response) and wait quietly. As it is usually hard to weep and talk at the same time, you might want to leave this until after it has passed or until the end of the hands-on part of the session. Meanwhile, you can consult yourself to see if you have an idea of the cause, or you can simply get on with what you were doing until either they initiate something or there is a good time. Depending on the type of crying – the tears are falling quietly, it is impossible to stop, the client is embarrassed by it, or the weeping is severe and causing so much distress that they are moving around – your response will vary. Acknowledgement and acceptance are key.

If you work a lot with those who are sad, you can choose to tell potential clients in advance that this might happen; mention it at the start of a session, or even put it on your website. Some like to be warned. Otherwise, you and they will manage the situation between you as it arises.

Forgiveness, apologies, thanks, goodbye

Asking for forgiveness for something we thought should not have been done or said, that we have reflected on and want to acknowledge with a client, is unusual in our work if we believe that whatever happens is *meant to be*. There may be times, though, when we do want to say sorry. Preparing in advance by reflecting and talking about it to someone else will be useful. Remember to assess the result afterwards and add to your client notes. It will change the power relationship between you.

There are many situations I have come across at the end of life when my clients are looking for forgiveness or wishing for an apology from others. If they have access to counselling, this may be a good place for them to go. Accepting your client and their story over a long period of time can make a difference. The Shiatsu diagnosis may reveal Lung's sadness which needs to be expressed, Large Intestine's function of letting go, Spleen's sense of the client's own self-blame, and so on.

The insurance broker Balens advises that apologizing is tantamount to admitting culpability and so should be considered carefully. Therefore, it depends on our relationship with our clients and the circumstances we find ourselves in. If you know or suspect that you have done something wrong, discuss it as soon as possible with a colleague or supervisor, then phone your insurance company and discuss it with them. They like to know before the official complaint comes in.

We thank our clients because we have been trusted with their bodymind and learned from the opportunity. If they die before we next see them, this will be good for our healing process. If they do not come back for other reasons, there will be a sense of completion.

Saying goodbye is instinctive. Once we have laid our hands on someone who is dying, we will know that, and wishing them well on their journey, wherever we feel they are going, is a way of acknowledging what we both know. I turned at the door to take a last look at a client and we smiled at each other. She said, 'I'll be seeing you.'

— Chapter 7 —

For Teachers, Students and Postgraduate Practitioners

For teachers

I hope that this book will be useful for teachers who want to include death and loss as topics either in their undergraduate or postgraduate training programmes. Please note that although this chapter covers areas which are particularly appropriate to the teaching situation, there is information in the other chapters which might also be helpful, specifically Chapter 5, The Practitioner.

Teaching about death and loss

Death and loss arise inevitably and naturally when we practise Shiatsu professionally, but new students will not have come across it unless facing it directly in their personal lives or unless they have specialist knowledge in this area, without Shiatsu, such as bereavement counselling, working as a social worker with a particular group, or for a charity, like Marie Curie Cancer Care.

As teachers, we want to give our students adequate preparation for their clinic work. The topics we choose to add to the basic curriculum are probably related to our own experience and expertise, to what students have requested, or what we believe is a well-rounded education. We may offer elective subjects or advanced clinical applications, maybe inviting visiting teachers to cover them during the undergraduate programme or afterwards. This section offers ways to introduce death and loss to your students at various levels.

Death and loss within the curriculum

Working with death and loss can be a stand-alone subject or part of another one(s) such as practice management (the practicalities of managing your practice and how you deal with clients) or counselling and listening skills (this topic addresses open listening and acceptance in the therapeutic scenario).

First and foremost, as teachers, it is important to spend some personal time on this topic. Your aim as a teacher is to find out how you personally want to tackle the subject in class, and why:

- Reading is one form of continuing professional development/ education and there are many suggestions in the Further Reading and Resources section at the back of the book.

- If this type of work is not a speciality, then a second form of continuing professional development/education – in fact your primary resource – is your client notes. Notes from sessions with people who were grieving, facing a life-threatening illness or at the end of life will give you plenty of examples to inspire and educate your students in class.

- Courses run by a local organization specializing in this area could offer training and support. This would include bereavement training through an organization like Cruse[1] in the UK or Griefline[2] in Australia, which both offer a telephone helpline to those who are needing support with the grieving process. There may be training through the local hospital or hospice where you work.

- Perhaps you could go somewhere to talk with, and listen to, those who deal with people in these situations, such as other health professionals, spiritual leaders, death doulas (O'Brien 2017), or undertakers.

- There may be a specific Shiatsu group or continuing professional development/education course which focuses on this topic, where you can get ideas and share experiences.

---

1   Cruse Bereavement Care, England, Ireland and Wales: www.cruse.org.uk; Scotland: www.crusescotland.org.uk
2   https://griefline.org.au

Formulating your aim and method

What moves you about this subject? The focus of your lesson plan can reflect some of the memories and lessons learned from your own life, your client work and the activities listed above. In addition, you will have a sense of what you appreciated from your own Shiatsu training. Then you can start to formulate what you would like to present to your students.

I remember the meditation Suzanne Yates led on the first weekend of her Wellmother (Yates 1990) training many years ago. We were directed into our pelvis, into the uterus itself, and imagined our own birth. The beginning of life rather than death, yes, but as a teaching tool it was very effective in taking us right to the heart of the matter and ensuring we were engaged both viscerally and emotionally with the subject at hand. From its website, I see that the Zen Caregiving Project[3] in San Francisco invites those on its programme to do a similar thing, to imagine their death.

There are generally two main parts to the death and loss part of a student training programme:

- Student self-development

- Preparation for working with clients who are facing death in some way.

Student self-development

What do students need to know to create a safe environment for themselves and their practice clients? What skills will they need as practitioners?

Below I have outlined the areas of a baseline curriculum (from the CNHC Guidelines UK) which include aspects of the death and loss topic.

The theoretical frameworks relevant to the safe and appropriate delivery of bodywork

It may be useful to examine the place of death in the theoretical frameworks you teach to your students in order that they have a basic understanding of how the underlying theory relates to it. For example, if

---

3   www.zenhospice.org

you teach the Five Elements, then you will study the connection between Metal, grief, sadness and melancholy. If you present TCM, then you will go into the function of Jing and how it depletes with age, bringing certain associations with it – dementia, loss of kidney function and so on.

- Medical anatomy, physiology and pathology (APP) in physical and mental health: In order to fully prepare students for clinical practice in this area, training must include both basic APP and research skills. It is useful for them to be able to understand and work with the medical diagnosis and prognosis, common and current medications, and basic hospital procedures as they relate to the client's complications near death.

- Shiatsu practice: To be able to assess, and then discuss, when Shiatsu is appropriate or not with the client, their family and other health professionals.

- General wellbeing: To be able to recognize a state of general wellbeing and deviations from that, what Shiatsu is appropriate in the case of said deviations, and why someone would want it (that is, what is the difference between Western and Eastern models of healthcare, what do clients learn from Shiatsu?).

- Improvements: To be able to recognize and discuss the client's health and effective functioning on all four levels regarding death and loss.

- Short-term client reactions (grief and day-to-day loss): To be able to recognize and discuss the ongoing and/or intensification of symptoms or reactions in the short term.

- Maintenance and stability: To be able to offer appropriate recommendations for maintaining client health and stability, after and between sessions.

- Basic counselling and listening skills: To be able to apply these to the particularities of grief and loss and, where required, to avoid common practitioner–client relational concerns, such as control and power issues which arise when negotiating the client's own religious beliefs or cultural differences.

- Limitations: To recognize the limitations of one's own knowledge, skills and experience, and the importance of not exceeding them.

- Support and self-care: To be able to support emotional expression or release for the client and as a practitioner.

- Practice management: To be able to understand the framework of privacy and confidentiality, note-taking skills, and safety. Basic administration, such as drawing up a contract with a client who has cancer.

- Health and safety: To be able to carry out a risk assessment, to identify when it is appropriate to give Shiatsu bodywork.

- Contraindications: To be able to recognize contraindications which pertain to grief and end-of-life care.

- Palliative care: To be able to define palliative care, the places where it is offered and by whom, its aims, how the Shiatsu practitioner interacts with other professionals and patients, and possible outcomes.

- Session evaluation: To be able to assess the session(s) from the practitioner and client's perspective by using appropriate methods, measures and gauges. This includes research methods for collating and assessing data.

Preparation for working with clients who are facing death

Students need the impetus and time to think about what death means to them. We do not always readily face death, not if it brings sadness and distress into our day. It can be an emotive subject, so care must be taken to think through and prepare the class, allowing for adequate space and support, including student follow-up on a one-to-one basis if necessary.

You can choose to give them warning that the topic will be covered and when. If it is a compulsory part of the undergraduate programme, you might want to explain why you think it is important and are covering it with them. Alternatively, you can start the session by asking them why they think it is being covered. For some, the notification will be enough to prompt thought, discussion and/or writing. For others, it will cause worry or upset in advance, and it may be appropriate to allow class time to express this. It is useful to notice who does not attend the session and to follow up afterwards in case they are needing some help. You may also want to cover it with them privately or set some homework to be done instead.

Sample exercises

Title: Introduction to Working with Death and Loss for the Shiatsu Practitioner.

Aim: To stimulate a discussion about death and loss in Shiatsu practice, and start to identify particular ways of working with this client group.

Creating a safe space: It is important to set up a safe place where the members of the group can focus and express their ideas and feelings about death, without judgement or embarrassment. A meditation circle around a candle (with its connotations of a shrine or memorial), or a Chi Gung exercise such as The Gathering of Essence and Shen from Chapter 8, are two suggestions.

Journal work: Private journal writing in a class setting would ordinarily come after an exercise, as a way of consolidating, inviting the student to reflect on what he has just done, on anything he has learned, and to make notes for the future, based on tutor support and personal reflection. With death and loss, it may be useful to offer some quiet time alone at the start. This will give the student the chance to remember and, importantly, to choose what and what not to share. Memories involving death and loss are almost always intense, and as this is a class rather than a therapeutic session, this might be necessary.

Questions you can pose for journal work: What experiences have you had with death, a) personally, and b) in your life outside Shiatsu?

Exercise 1

Choose a timescale – perhaps 5–15 minutes for each person. Ask the students to pair up – one lies down or sits in a position of her choice, and the other sits beside her. Tell the students to take time to settle, and when it seems right, use one hand to touch somewhere. Once contact has been made, they must be still and present, and notice what arises for them. Other than adjusting in the case of discomfort (changing position or adding a cushion, for example), the students must try to stay with the one touch. Then they swap over. Give time for them to write down their responses afterwards.

Exercise 2

Use some basic questions and/or some Clean Language:

1. *How are you today?*

2. Using the key word from their reply, say: *And is there anything else about...x?*

3. Follow the answer to this with another question: *And is there anything else about...x?*

4. Ask: *If this session could be exactly what you need, what would that be like?*

5. As well as repeating their words, notice their gesture and movement.

6. To get clear instructions about the Shiatsu your partner wants, say: *And to...(answer to Question 4), what would you like to have happen?*

7. You can use more Clean Language or other questions to make sure you are clear about what the receiver would like in order to meet his aim.

8. Give your partner ten minutes of the Shiatsu which he has asked for. Do not make your own choice; do exactly what he asked.

9. At the end, refer back to what they asked for and sum up: *And you said that a session which would be exactly what you needed would be...x. How was it?*

10. Swap over.

For example:

1. 'How are you today?' *I am tired.*

2. 'And is there anything else about tired?' *My mind is tired out.*

3. 'And is there anything else about "My mind is tired out"?' *It stops me making decisions.*

4. 'If this session could be exactly what you need, what would that be like?' *I would feel refreshed and know what to do.*

5. Repeat 'I would feel refreshed and know what to do' (with gesture/movement).

6. 'And to feel refreshed and know what to do, what would you like to have happen?' *Something on my back...and the sides of my head.* 'And what kind of back...and sides of your head Shiatsu would you like?' *Firm.*

7. 'And is there anything else about firm Shiatsu on your back and sides of your head?' *Firm...and kindly.* 'Firm and kindly Shiatsu on your back and sides of your head to feel refreshed and know what to do.'

8. Give your partner ten minutes of the Shiatsu which they have asked for. Do not make your own choice; do exactly what they asked.

9. 'And you said that a session which would be exactly what you needed would be refreshing, so that you would know what to do. How was it?' *I don't feel so tired and it was strange, but in the middle, I had an idea about what I could do.*

Exercise 3

1. Listen to your partner tell you how she is.

2. Sit quietly beside your partner and tune in. Take in all the information you need using your eyes, smell, taste and your own internal sensations, but do not ask any questions or do a touch diagnosis as a method of making a plan.

3. Give your partner ten minutes of Shiatsu using your intuition. It may be that you do nothing except sit beside them or make one simple touch. The receiver must say if there is something which causes them pain or which makes them feel bad, otherwise they are silent throughout.

4. Swap over.

Self-reflection questions
For receivers:

• In exercise 1, how did you feel about the simple touch?

- In exercise 2, how did you feel about asking for what you wanted?

- In exercise 3, how did you feel about what your partner did?

- Which of the three exercises did you prefer?

For givers:

- In exercise 1, how was sitting still with the one touch?

- In exercise 2, how was it to rely on your partner's instructions?

- In exercise 3, how did you feel about taking the initiative?

- Which of the three exercises did you prefer?

For everyone:

- How do these three exercises relate to situations in which your client is facing death?

- Does the client know what she wants?

- Do you feel confident in such circumstances?

Points to discuss in the big group afterwards

Exercise 1: We are hoping for feedback about how it feels to give and receive a very simple touch. There will be a range of responses, perhaps some receivers who felt they wanted more than that, and others who felt they had the support and freedom to become aware of themselves without interference from the practitioners. There are times at the end of life when this is either the only way or seems to be the best way to make contact with the client, to say, 'I am here, listening', while letting them focus on their internal state.

It is also useful to hear from the givers, whether they were comfortable with being still, on all four levels, or whether it raised some issues for them.

Exercise 2: It can be useful for the client to decide what they want if they have symptoms the practitioner is unfamiliar with; if they are in extreme pain; if they have control issues; if they doubt Shiatsu; or cannot trust the practitioner for whatever reason. It can be good for clients to learn to identify and ask for what they want. At the end of life or in grief, people can feel that the time is short or that they are very sensitive, and it can sometimes help if they are making the decisions and directing the practitioner. It is never too late for someone to learn more about themselves and their needs, where and how they want to be touched. Some or all of these points may be raised as a result of the student's reflections and responses, and, of course, there may be others too.

Exercise 3: It can be useful for the practitioner to decide what to do if the client is in an extreme situation, if they have not had Shiatsu before, or if they are too ill to know what they want. Once again, some or all of these points may be raised as a result of the student's reflections and responses, and, of course, there may be others too.

Practical exercise

See the section entitled 'The Po and the Hun' in Chapter 2 for more information about these aspects if need be. First, try the exercise with yourself and a colleague to ascertain your own reactions. See Table 7.1 for the location of the Tsubos.

Table 7.1: Tsubos associated with death and loss: BL 42 (Po) and BL 47 (Hun)

Tsubo name	Meridian location	Tsubo location	Physical location	Tsubo function
BL 42 (*Pohu*) for the Po	On the Secondary Bladder meridian	Adjacent to the LU Yu (Shu) BL 13 (Feishu)	Three cun lateral to the posterior midline between thoracic 3 and 4	Depending on the diagnosis, to calm or vitalize the Corporeal Spirit
BL 47 (*Hunmen*) for the Hun	On the Secondary Bladder meridian	Adjacent to the LV Yu (Shu) BL 18 (Ganshu)	Three cun lateral to the posterior midline between thoracic 9 and 10	Depending on the diagnosis, to anchor or release the Ethereal Spirit

Maciocia (1989) gives us (Secondary) Bladder points for each of the Treasures and they provide a way for students to make a first-hand acquaintance with them. Ask them to all sit or lie supine, comfortably, and take them through a guided meditation. There may be several layers of awareness – the physical (of the muscles and local sensation); emotional (sadness, melancholy); mental (consciousness of separation and boundaries); and spiritual (connection, via the Air Ki and Blood, to mortality, life and death). Traditionally, the Secondary Bladder points have more of a connection to the emotional aspect of the element or meridian than the Yu (Shu) points, which are more physical and sense organ related.

BL 42

1. Take your attention to your Bladder 42 Tsubos. Reach the right arm over the opposite shoulder, hold on to the right elbow to increase the stretch. With the fingers of the right hand, count down from the seventh cervical vertebrae to the depression inferior to the spinous process of thoracic 3 and, laterally, to just inside the medial edge of the scapula to find Bladder 42.

2. Use your right forefinger if possible (Large Intestine finger, most connected to Lung), or middle one if not, to activate the Tsubo.

3. Move your left arm laterally, hand in line with the shoulder, so you can feel the trapezius and rhomboideus muscles moving. There may be referred physical awareness in the neck. Now replace the left hand on the right elbow for support if you need it.

4. Notice what is happening in your chest. Notice if your breathing is affected.

5. Take your attention to your diaphragm and the solar plexus area. Make a mental note of anything that you feel there.

6. Finally, what is happening in your head and the rest of your body? (You might want to reassure that a 'spacey' feeling is them making a connection with the Blood.)

7. After some time (five minutes, perhaps), repeat on the other side.

BL 47

Ask the students to pair up. One lies in prone or sits and the other locates and connects with Bladder 47 on both sides of the spine simultaneously (see Figure 7.1), maintaining the contact for up to five minutes each. Swap over. Afterwards, give them time to write down what they noticed as both givers and receivers.

Have a group sharing and discussion about the exercise.

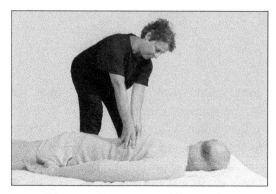

FIGURE 7.1: WORKING BLADDER 47 (*HUNMEN*) FOR THE HUN

Extend the class and/or discussion to use these Tsubos to diagnose and treat in the clinical setting. It is also beneficial to harmonize the two acupoints together: Bladder 42 and Bladder 47 on one side, and then both of them on the other side.

Working BL 42 and BL 47 in the side position – three possibilities

- Try using your left hand to do all four points (middle finger on the spine, forefinger and thumb on the two points on the right side of the client's back and ring finger and little pinkie finger covering the two points on the left side of the client's back) while the Mother hand rests on the hip.

- Work BL 42 and BL 47 with each of your thumbs on the upper side of the client's back and, when he turns over, repeat on the other side. If it is not possible for the infirm client to roll over, one side will be sufficient.

- It is possible to thumb both BL 42 points at the same time using two hands if you can enable your Hara to be low enough when working on a futon, but it will be easier on a hospital bed because it is higher up and you can sit on a chair or stool to be comfortable.

Working BL 42 and BL 47 in the supine position – two possibilities

- Slide your hand(s) under the client's back and activate by levering up (contraindication: this may be uncomfortable for the client if she has any pain or bedsores).

- Place a hand on the client's body, preferably above the points, and use your imagination to activate the Tsubos with your thoughts and intention.

Working BL 42 and BL 47 in the prone position

It is straightforward to work these Tsubos in prone if your client can lie comfortably in that position.

Whichever position you choose, remember to keep an awareness of your own BL 42 and BL 47 Tsubos as you connect with those of your client, for a deeper and more powerful effect if that is required.

Tutor reflection practice

- Did I enjoy teaching the session about death?

- Was I happy with the way it went?

- What are my learning points?

- Would I do anything differently next time?

Working with students who are facing death

You may have students in your group who are close to someone who is dying or has died, or who have received a serious or life-threatening diagnosis.

A student is close to someone who is dying

It is not unusual for a student to be dealing with a dying relative, close friend or pet, and subsequently to be grieving. Of course, there is no reason why she should not remain in the school, although if it is debilitating or she is absent for more than two weekends, you may want to suggest that she takes a temporary break and returns the following year. It is also possible that the student who is managing this will speak at length in the opening circle and this might have to be curtailed or a private conversation had with the person concerned if she is diverting the group's focus.

A student is close to death

Here is a basic scenario: The student either speaks directly to you or sends you a message with the news. You speak with the student to get the full picture and to understand her feelings and approach. She wants to remain in the group, explaining why. You discuss it with your colleagues (fellow teachers and assistants) and debate the possibilities and outcomes, how you might deal with them and whether it will disrupt the group more than educate them. You decide if you accept this, and write down your response, followed by informing the student of your decision, together with any provisos. For example, it is likely that you will need to be kept up to date with the student's progress, perhaps there will be a discussion with their consultant, maybe with the family. You will need contact details and to go over what to do in an emergency. All teachers and assistants will need to be informed.

You advise the student that you support her telling the rest of the group, and discuss when and how. You make time in the weekend plan for that. You devise a way for feedback and questions, perhaps telling them on the Saturday evening (if you have a weekend course) so they can think about it overnight and then revisiting the topic on Sunday morning, or as appropriate. You make a statement about the school's response and what you hope will happen, such as: 'We will support x, encouraging her to be a working member of the group as much as is possible and ensuring that the lessons are not disrupted. She will update everyone in the opening circle each Saturday morning (or at the beginning of the class), so that those of you who are pairing up with her will know what to expect and so that she does not have to tell each one of you individually, as she is hoping to get on with her life and studying without focusing on it all the time.'

Being in the group may be supportive to the student who is dying or has a life-threatening diagnosis. It will be a learning experience for the others, both for themselves and their future client work. Some may be distressed and you may choose to spend time with them or with anyone who is opposed to her remaining.

There may be situations where health and safety measures must be taken to protect the group and individual, but when dealt with appropriately, it is a great education for everyone concerned. An example of this would be having a student who is HIV positive. Privacy for the person concerned and safety for the group must be debated, and it will be an opportunity for the other students to attain a thorough understanding of the condition and of what care must be taken with clients.

There may be a time when you decide it is impossible to continue to work with a student. As inclusion is enshrined in the Equalities Act (Europe), you will have to give well-thought-out reasons for this (perhaps the others' learning is compromised because of a mental health condition where the individual is unstable). If this is the case, you may want to take advice from your professional association, colleagues in other schools, the school insurance company and others.

If a student chooses to leave, it is recommended that they communicate this to the rest of the group themselves. We all know how intimate the group becomes when they are studying together, and changes to the make-up of it are usually significant. There will probably need to be time set aside to allow for reactions from those left.

Working with the rest of the group when one of them is dying
If you have been integrating a dying student and she becomes unable to continue, the reactions may be complex:

- Grief at her absence – sadness and missing the contribution she made to the class.

- Blame and guilt – what if we did something wrong? Did we do enough to help?

- Fear for one's own death – what if I die too, after all I am a bit similar to her and we were interested in the same things? Is there a connection between learning Shiatsu and death? (We can be very irrational at such times.)

- Anger – she was such a great person, why did she have to die?

See Chapter 3 for more information on this aspect.

Funerals and memorials
If the student concerned has died, then there will be a need for grieving and forming a new group identity. It may be that there is a funeral or memorial and that members of the group want to attend. Activities that the student was an integral part of (a joint project, a buddy for another student in the same or another year, for example) will have to

be rethought, and this will have an impact. Even something like turning a previously even-numbered group into an odd-numbered one will make a difference.

The announcement of the death of TD, one of my former students, came just before the annual residential in the Scottish countryside. It was being held in the same venue as the previous year when she had been with us. Her funeral was being held while we were there. We debated whether to leave and attend, and instead the group carried out their own Shiatsu-style memorial in the garden. We spoke about her and our memories of her and made a fitting ritual for the occasion. It was, of course, very moving and we had to make time around it out of respect, to grieve and start the integration stage – we had to find a way to move on without her. A place was left for her in the circle and she was often and appropriately remembered.

Another time we each lit a candle and sent them up into the night sky in paper lanterns. (This may not be considered environmentally friendly now.)

The choice to attend a student's funeral or memorial is an individual one and may depend on how long she had been training at your school.

Contacting the family, contributing to obituaries

This may apply to past students or current ones. You may want to contact her family and send your condolences and/or those of your school or group.

An obituary in the newsletter of your local or national professional association may also be requested. This would include:

- how you knew her – why you are writing it

- who she was – in general (brief) and in the Shiatsu context

- personal recollection(s) of the group/school

- any practical details – date of the memorial or a word or two about the event if it is in the past.

Your personal response: when someone dies there is often a gap in our lives (see Chapter 5, The Practitioner, 'Death of a colleague'). When it is a student we have cared for over time, there can be a sense that we feel like a parent to them. The bond between a teacher and a student is very strong. Not only were they learning a new skill from us which could have changed their lives, but we have engaged with their Ki (receiving from them, probably giving, helping them feel it, and identifying their learning style so that we can support them through the course). As with a client dying, this is a significant part of our life. So, as well as supporting the other students and acting in our professional capacity, we must remember to allow ourselves time to mourn alone, perhaps writing down some of our feelings, speaking to a colleague who also taught them, or working with a bereavement counsellor.

When we are grieving

If we are grieving, we may find that we are unable to plan the next class or make practical arrangements.

When my father died, I found a replacement teacher for the first class I was due to teach and she worked without a brief from me. However, as it got closer and closer to the second weekend, four weeks later, I found myself unable to mark homework, or make up a timetable – I could not think coherently. I had left it too late to cancel or find someone else, so, with support from my supervisor, I turned up, vulnerable, but reassured that I could manage one way or another. I sat in front of the class and began to explain what had happened to my father and I cried.

As the students realized that I had yielded control, they stepped forward and took it themselves. It was a Wood weekend and the year plan listed the meridians and Tsubos we would cover. The students had their files with the diagrams, and so they arranged things themselves, concluding that it was a great thing to do with this element because being controlled and having to follow a tight schedule can send Wood into imbalance. I was present, but in a different capacity. The students were fine, and it was a great learning process for us all.

For students and practitioners

If you are a student learning about death and loss, your teacher will have explained why this is part of your undergraduate training. You may have already come across these topics with your practice clients or in other parts of your life. Covering it in class will boost your confidence, raise your awareness and enable a good discussion with your colleagues.

If it has not been a unit on your course and you would like it to be, you can raise the subject with your tutor. It is not a specified part of most core curricula and has been traditionally dealt with as it arises when discussing case studies or the theory of the Five Elements and TCM. However, death and loss are being talked about much more nowadays, so it may be a topic that your school would consider covering, if you make a request.

You might be a practitioner with a special feeling for this work; you may want to gain further experience because you have a new position at a hospice or a care home; or you may simply welcome the chance of a more in-depth discussion about loss in the lives of your clients. Undertaking a postgraduate workshop or course may provide you with what you are looking for, or you could organize one for yourself and your colleagues.

Organizing a gathering to initiate such an idea is simple. Here are some ideas to get you started:

- You could initiate a Shiatsu practice class focusing on death and loss, or set aside a half-day for a workshop where you each take it in turns to present some Shiatsu which is relevant to death and loss.

- You could make an altar or shrine to someone or something (see Chapter 4 for information about making an altar).

- You could devise a ritual for saying goodbye to something which has had its time, or for this stage of your life (see Chapter 3 for information about rituals).

- You could hold a Death Cafe. This is a discussion-based event centred around tea and cake or a meal, where participants sit in small groups with a menu of discussion topics on the subject of death and loss. It is talk-and not touch-based. Everyone is there for the same reason and there is an emphasis on listening and sharing.

The focus is that life is finite. The family of the organizer of the first such event has made a website with full instructions. You can devise a menu to sit on the tables with a list of questions for discussion. Divided into starters (quickies such as 'Cremation or burial?'); mains (longer, more in-depth questions for consideration); and dessert, tea and coffee (lighter issues to end with, such as 'What song would you like at your funeral?'). They do not have to be proscriptive, but are there to keep the conversation moving. You can change tables between courses so that you are sitting next to someone different if you like. Sample questions include: 'Do you support nature taking its course or assisted suicide?', 'Where would you like to be when you die?', 'What words do you want on your tombstone?', 'Is there such a thing as a"good death"?' A true Death Cafe does not have a menu as above. If you want to use one, you will have to give your event another name.

> 'In the Death Cafe there are no hierarchies. We all meet simply as people who are going to die.' (Underwood 2011)

You could also host a discussion group. Consider the following points:

- How much time do you have for the discussion?

- How many people might attend?

- Choose the questions you want to discuss (allowing at least ten minutes per person per question as a basic guideline).

Here are some questions you can use to get your group started:

- Have you ever had to watch someone suffer? What was it like? What did it do to your Ki? What did you do?

- Do you think that children and adults feel the same way when someone has died? Do they need different sorts of support?

- Is loss the same for all of us?

- In what ways can we support ourselves to be able to do this sort of work?

You can also use these questions alone, in your co-counselling, supervision or peer-support groups (see Chapter 5). Undertaking these activities will count as continuing professional development/education, so include a record of what you did, why and what you discovered in your log book for the end of the year.

For more information on using rite and ritual in teaching or practice around death, see also Chapter 4.

— Chapter 8 —

Practical Exercises

This chapter contains exercises and meditations for you, the Shiatsu practitioner, if you want to work with the subjects of death and loss, and particularly with clients who are at the end of their life. The *Tao Te Ching* equates life with pliancy and death with rigidity ('So hardness and stiffness go with death; tenderness, softness, go with life') (Lao Tzu, trans. LeGuin 2011, p.110). Being still and holding positions are powerful ways to promote this quality of softness, awareness and an open attitude. Standing Like a Tree and other Qi gong, alongside meditation, can enable a flexible physical strength (to avoid injury), as well as a calm mental, emotional and spiritual stability which is necessary for this vital support.

Another aspect of being with dying or grieving clients which requires focus is that of boundaries. It is useful for practitioners to address and understand their boundaries when working in highly emotional or serious medical situations, and where the spirit is preparing to separate from the Corporeal Soul. This is not to say that we cannot share or feel, but knowing where our Ki meets the receiver's, and about our limitations, can be useful. Grounding can never be under-estimated, it is the root of our practice and our way to a greater connection.

Qi gong

If you can, practise Qi gong outside in a beautiful and peaceful place away from too much pollution. That way you are breathing clean, fresh air and the energy of nature will support you.

Standing in bare feet will allow you to make an even better connection with the earth, as long as you are warm enough. Being on a cold surface or doing it in autumn/winter can cause a chill to ascend, so follow your own instinct on this. There are scientists now looking at why a barefoot practice is beneficial, and it appears to be because electrons are being absorbed through Bubbling Spring (Yongquan Kidney 1). This makes sense to us! James Oschman states, "'Grounded' or 'earthed' means that our bodies are connected to earth's abundant supply of electrons. This is a natural condition in which earth's electrons spread over and into our bodies, stabilizing our internal electrical environment."[1]

Historically in China, Medical Qi gong doctors would focus on purging stagnant spiritual energy from the body in preparation for death. This is in line with clients' statements: that they want to clear out old memories, especially negative ones, say sorry or make amends. A personal Qi gong practice can enable an internal understanding of the benefits of such exercises and the practitioner can then teach or use them with clients where appropriate.

Standing Like a Tree

This is such a traditional part of Qi gong that if you have engaged with any sort of training before you have probably done this or another version. It is very simple and all forms are as valid and powerful as each other.

Note: With all breathing instructions, if your nose is blocked and you cannot breathe in and out of your nose, breathe the way that you can. It may be that the practice of these exercises will make it possible over time.

Wu Chi is often (but not always) symbolized by an empty circle, a never-ending line filled with apparent space (see Figure 8.1). Like the answer to 'Where exactly is that point?' and 'So, the meridian goes precisely where?', the essence of Zen eludes definition, defies grasping. It has connotations of the sky when it has cleared, the sound in your ears when you are underwater, the falling before sleep, simultaneously before-the-beginning and after-the-end.

---

1   Search for *The Human Story* on YouTube to find out more about his presentation to the Annual World Congress of Anti-Aging Medicine.

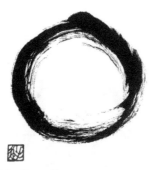

FIGURE 8.1: THE WU CHI – I AM INSEPARABLE FROM EVERYTHING

Here is quite precise guidance on taking the Wu Chi stance (see Figure 8.2) so that you can experience the empty circle! Stand with your feet hip-width apart or slightly wider if that feels more stable. Your toes are facing forwards and your heels back, lining up the insteps along imaginary straight lines. Visualize roots growing down from Bubbling Spring (Yongquan Kidney 1) into the earth, with relaxed knees as if your patellae are moving forwards and over your middle toes. If you think about the fact that your coccyx points forwards, you will find that your pelvis gently tilts in the same direction without having to make a big adjustment. Imagine the Tsubo which is the Gate of Life (Ming Men GV or Du 4 between lumbar vertebrae 3 and 4) opening. Your arms are hanging loosely, palms towards the sides of your thighs, and there is air under your armpits so you can breathe easily into the seams of your body. Your shoulder blades are slipping down your back, there is some space in the joint between your mandible and maxilla, and the tip of your tongue is touching the red of the roof of your mouth behind the top teeth. It is as if you are suspended from a silver thread originating in the heavens. Your eyes are open and looking, with a soft gaze, just below the horizon.

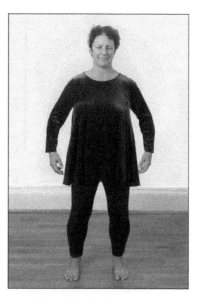

FIGURE 8.2: THE WU CHI STANCE – QUIET TIME
BEFORE AND AFTER MOVEMENT

Focus on your breath. Follow it as it passes in and out of your nostrils, soundlessly.

On an outbreath, an exhalation, very slowly and mindfully raise your arms forward until they are about shoulder height. Ensure that your shoulders do not rise and close the Gallbladder 21 area off to the Ki. Your arms are gently curved, with palms towards the centre of your chest. Your elbows are at least as high as your hands or a little higher (as if a drop of water would roll down your forearms and off your forefingers), with your fingertips facing each other. The space between your middle fingertips is about two inches (four centimetres). Inhale. Exhale (see Figure 8.3).

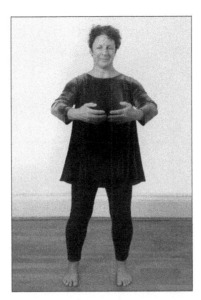

FIGURE 8.3: STANDING LIKE A TREE

Start to inhale and let that incoming breath be your impetus for opening the arms to the sides, allowing your shoulders to stay in a relaxed state, palms and insides of elbows facing front, and making sure you can still see your fingers out of the corners of your eyes.

You are a tree! Keep standing; send your roots down and out. Breathe in, breathe out, and repeat. Every now and then check your posture, making micro-adjustments of your arms, hands and fingers (branches, leaves and pine needles) if necessary, and your mind for thoughts (flowers and fruit), although the general aim is to be still and not to think. You are aware of your surroundings, but not engaged with them. You notice your thoughts and feelings, but are not distracted by them.

The mantra is 'I am not' (see Figure 8.4).

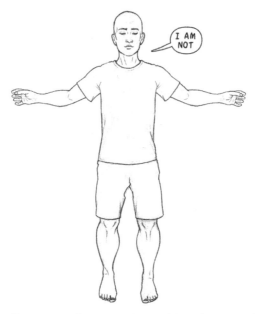

FIGURE 8.4: STANDING LIKE A TREE: 'I AM NOT'

Variations:

- Allow your arms to move ever so slightly with your breath as if the wind is moving them, or as if a bird has landed on you.

- Open them to the sides of you, so that you can still see your hands in your peripheral vision and your palms are facing front, but elbows and shoulders are in the same configuration.

- Keep your arms in the same shape they were in when they were ahead of you, but transfer them upwards until they are in front of your forehead, raising your eyeballs to look in that direction.

How long to stay in the pose? The traditional way is to start with five minutes a day for a week and see how you get on, lengthening your practice to six minutes for the second week, then seven minutes and so on. Some people do it for an hour or more, regularly.

What are the benefits?

- Your temperature will probably change – warming if you tend to be cool, and vice versa.

- Your Ki and muscular strength will increase. The Ki is meant to build up inside you, so do not shake it off or out unless it feels best.

- Your patience will also probably increase.

- You are likely to feel more peaceful (after a while).

- It will give you a break from everyday life.

If parts of you hurt, your legs start to shake or you have strong feelings, you can try to:

- really notice what is happening

- take a deeper breath

- relax the shaking or painful part

- try staying with the sensation – it will eventually change

- come out of the pose slowly, stretch, and come back another time

- let yourself be moved for a while, for the life in you to express itself.

Do not push yourself, there is enough time to get used to this and to deepen your practice!

Note: Throughout the exercises, pay attention to your wrists and other joints, adjusting placement and position to keep them relaxed and comfortable at all times. You might need to experiment with this until you have found a way to follow the exercise without strain.

Qi gong for the Lungs

This exercise is perhaps the one I find myself using the most in my work with those who are grieving and dying. So many people have chronic obstructive pulmonary disease, lung cancer or other breathing issues that it is a really useful exercise to have in your 'toolbox'. It is so beautifully simple and can be performed in a chair or standing, lying supine. You can teach it to your client who can even do it, privately, in a hospital lavatory cubicle if they are shy. It is very helpful if done on top of a hill or by the sea for the purity of Ki and air.

Take the Wu Chi stance and breathe smoothly. After a while, bring your arms and hands up to chest height, as if you are hugging a great oak as above. Your palms face your chest.

Inhale and let the breath which fills your lungs be the impetus for your arms to open, thumbs leading, palms upwards, like doors opening to the sides of you. See your hands in your peripheral vision at the same time as looking ahead. Don't let the arms open so much that you cannot see them (in other words do not overstretch the chest. The shoulder blades hardly come together at the back). This movement lasts for the length of that inhalation. Picture a great swan standing up on the water and flapping its white wings.

Exhale and join the thumbs and forefingers together on each hand, slowly folding your elbows and bringing the hands towards Lung 1 (but not quite touching the chest) (see Figure 8.5); unfold the elbows once more, palms down, opening the fingers back to the beginning position. Overall, it is a very subtle and gentle exercise. There should be no strain or sense of stretching at all. It is an internal energy exercise.

I recommend repeating five times every morning. There is no need to do more for the first few weeks but afterwards it can be increased if desired. Regularity of practice is key.

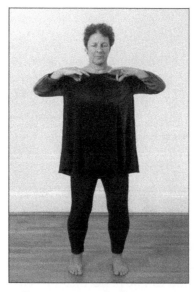

FIGURE 8.5: EXHALE TOWARDS LUNG 1 ON THE CHEST

The Gathering of Essence and Shen

This short exercise can:

- calm your Ki, so you can concentrate and connect

- boost your Ki, energizing you for the work ahead or if you are tired

- move your Ki, to rebalance and circulate, particularly to the hands, thumbs and fingers

- ground your Ki, positioning yourself between heaven and earth ready to give Shiatsu

- help you learn to control and focus the amount of oxygen and Air Ki that you take in and expel, to aid the above.

It can be done:

- once, as a quick way to prepare yourself

- as many times as you enjoy, so that you no longer have to think about the moves and breath, but can allow yourself to relax and meditate

- before a treatment, to make the transition from what you were doing before, to the sessions which are about to start

- afterwards, to come back to yourself and assess how you are, allowing any necessary letting go, observing issues which have arisen and need further exploration, or prepare for the next thing you are going to do.

For sound information on acupoints/acupressure points, please refer to the mobile phone Tsubook application: www.tsubook.net/en.

Preparation:

- Take the Wu Chi stance as above (Figure 8.2).

- Lay one palm on the Dantian (centre of the Hara around the Sea of Qi (Qihai Conception Vessel or Ren 6)) and the other one on top of it (Figure 8.6.1).

- Look forwards and slightly down with a soft gaze.
- Breathe gently.

Note: Other than the beginning and end positions, the palms do not touch the body but are a couple of inches (four to five centimetres) away from it.

The exercise is outlined in Table 8.1.

Table 8.1: The Gathering of Essence and Shen exercise

	Breathing *The breath initiates all movement*	Movements *The movement flows in response to, and alongside, your breath, smoothly and continuously, as if through clouds*
1	Breathing in	• (Please refer to Figure 8.6.2.) Open your arms out to the sides of your body, at a level between the waist and the shoulders and parallel to the ground, thumbs leading, palms upwards, shoulders relaxed, seeing both hands in your peripheral vision. • (Please refer to Figure 8.6.3.) Bring your palms towards your kidneys, not touching, and appreciate their warmth.
2	Breathing out	• (Please refer to Figure 8.6.4.) Move your palms past your sacrum and down the backs of your legs (covering the Large Intestine, Kidney, Lung, Bladder, Heart meridians/Zen extensions) until they are behind your heels, bending the knees as you do this and relaxing the back of your neck. • Start to turn your palms towards the earth and move your hands around the outside edges of your feet and past the ends of your toes. • (Please refer to Figure 8.6.5.) Imagine you are scooping up palmfuls of the earth's Ki.

3	Breathing in	• (Please refer to Figure 8.6.6.) Draw your palms along the insteps of your feet and up the Yin aspects of your legs (Heart, Kidney, Heart Governor, Small Intestine, Spleen Pancreas, Liver meridians/Zen extensions) to your Hara. • (Please refer to Figure 8.6.7.) Carry on moving your hands upwards, pointing your fingertips slightly towards the midline, moving up the centre of your torso (tracing the Conception Vessel or Ren channel) and tracing the profile of your face (Conception Vessel or Ren and Governing Vessel or Du channels) all the way to the top of your head, the *Place of 100 Meetings* (Governing Vessel or Du 20) at the crown chakra.
4	Breathing out	• (Please refer to Figure 8.6.8.) Open your palms upwards, look up, allow your throat to open, and appreciate the sky (or if inside, imagine it!). • Keep opening your naturally curved arms to the sides of your body until your elbows are about shoulder level and your hands a little higher.
5	Breathing in	• (Please refer to Figure 8.6.9.) Reverse that part by raising your arms up again until your palms are over the top of your head, the *Place of 100 Meetings* (Governing Vessel or Du 20, crown chakra), relaxing your neck so that the back of it is straight again.
6	Breathing out	• (Please refer to Figure 8.6.10.) With fingertips leading, draw a line down, mimicking the central vessel at the front of your face and body, but not touching, until they are level with your heart.
7	Breathing in	• (Please refer to Figure 8.6.11.) Trace a large heart shape in the air in front of your chest by moving the fingertips up towards your chin and outwards from each other, in a sweeping curve in front of the shoulders, downwards and towards each other to a point level with *Great Tower Gate* (Ju Que, Conception Vessel or Ren 14, Heart Bo or Mu point).
8	Breathing out	• (Please refer to Figure 8.6.1 (again).) You can end by replacing your hands one on top of each other on the Dantian and Hara. • Or you can repeat four more timees, or as many times as you like, beginning again at step one.

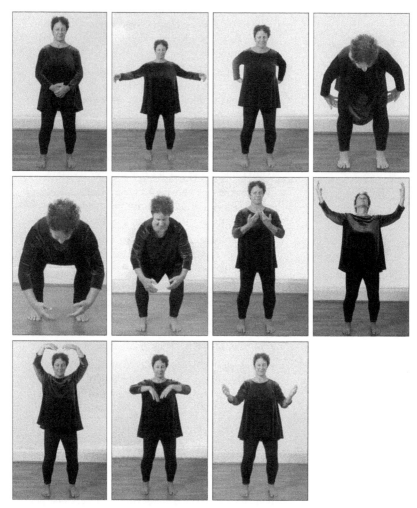

FIGURES 8.6.1–8.6.11: THE GATHERING OF ESSENCE AND SHEN

The mantra is 'I give and I am replenished' (see Figure 8.7).

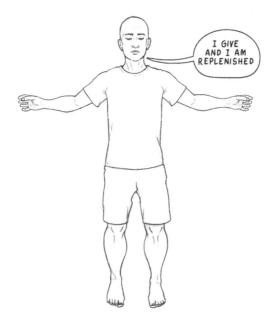

FIGURE 8.7: 'I GIVE AND I AM REPLENISHED'

Guided meditations

If you have not meditated before because you find, like I did, that you cannot sit still for five minutes, but want to try, here is an idea: start by getting to know what sort of environment you need to be able to concentrate, find a place and time where and when you will not be disturbed, and experiment with sitting or kneeling positions until you find one that is comfortable. Then try simply sitting still for *one* minute a day. Just one minute, without moving. Do not extend the time, stick to one minute every day for the first week. It might be surprising, but one week will make a difference. Keep a note of what happens each time and anything else noticeable that happens at other times. If you need some extra support, arrange to have Shiatsu until your practice is established. It will help with what arises and gets in the way, and give you some encouragement.

If you like it, try up to five minutes a day during week two and ten minutes in week three, or devise an alternative schedule that works for you. Joining a group can be easier than managing on your own. As you know from being in workshops, the collective Ki is very powerful and will be a great help. Alternatively, you could take a meditation or mindfulness course to launch your meditation practice.

Meditation is a way to:

- practise physically sitting still for varying lengths of time
- train the mind
- focus on your breath
- develop patience
- develop acceptance
- develop compassion
- connect with the four levels and seven chakras
- prepare for whatever arises between you and your client
- settle down after a session and separate from what has happened, taking space and time to re-energize for what will ensue.

Separating and Refining Meditation A

Aim: To recognize and strengthen your boundaries.

If you are not already an experienced meditator, take your time and gradually build up your ability to focus and breathe deeply in this way. If at any moment you feel uncomfortable physically, then mindfully and slowly adjust, or stop and start again after a stretch or a break. If it is an internal discomfort, perhaps you feel that you are hyperventilating or getting light headed – neither of these things are dangerous at this stage, but it is important that you notice and respect yourself by doing something about it right away. Do not push yourself, as there is enough time to get used to this and to deepen your practice.

This is a guided meditation and therefore you are less likely to be aware of random thoughts or niggling worries while you are doing it, but they will probably still find their way in. When this happens, look at them, recognize them as an old friend, smile and then turn away, back to your breathing and the images.

Preparation: Sit or kneel, cross legged or in seiza (see Figure 8.8), with or without a chair, stool or cushion(s), finding a position and place which allows your spine to be straight – coccyx down to the earth and crown to the heavens, and your mind at peace. Rest your hands on a cushion if you like, as it can be very supportive for your shoulders. Your eyes can be closed or open.

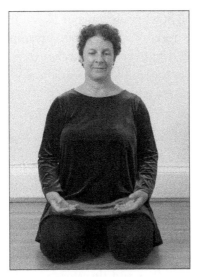

FIGURE 8.8: SEIZA

Lightly observe how you are today (that is, scan yourself): your body, feelings, thoughts and spiritual state, as if you are sitting in a beam of light which moves over and through you from top to toe collecting information or data about you in that instant. Do this lightly because it will not be useful in this context to attach any judgement to however you are, or make any changes to it unless they happen naturally and without effort, such as sitting up a bit straighter. Do all this mindfully so that you will have a residual memory of yourself for later comparison.

1. Notice your breathing: the air coming in and out of your nostrils, cool as it enters and warmer as it leaves.

2. Follow the route the air takes in through your nose and down your throat; then out through your nose, away from you, spreading and merging with the air in front of your face. It is as if you were outside on a cold night and you could see your breath crystallize as it disperses. Repeat this a few times.

3. Follow the air deeper: in through your nose and down your throat and expanding your whole chest (in three dimensions); out through your nose, away from you, spreading, merging with the air and dispersing over towards the wall, tree or something in front of you. Repeat this a few times.

4. Follow the air deeper still: in through your nose and down your throat, expanding your chest, pushing your diaphragm down

and filling the bowl made by your Hara, hips and sacrum; out through your nose, away from you, spreading, merging with the air, dispersing over towards the wall, tree or something in front of you, out over the land and up into the sky like a gentle swirling mist. Repeat this a few times.

5. Follow the air deeper and deeper: in through your nose and down your throat, expanding your chest, pushing your diaphragm down and filling the bowl of your Hara and sacrum; this time wait here, no movement in or out, no thoughts in the emptiness of your being. Feel the air naturally starting to flood back out through your nose, away from you, spreading, merging with the air, dispersing over towards the wall, tree or something in front of you, out over the land and up into the sky like a gentle swirling mist; and wait again, your attention and therefore your Ki out over the hills and mountains and among the trees in the forests, the fish in the ocean and the clouds in the sky, until the air naturally flows back in. Repeat this a few times. Never strain yourself uncomfortably, always allow yourself to respond to any unpleasant sensations by gently stopping and relaxing. See Figures 8.9 and 8.10.

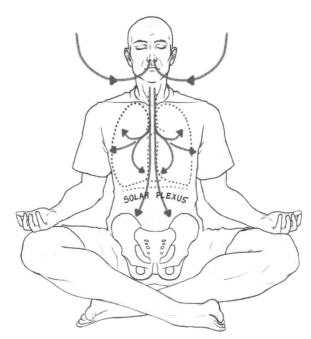

FIGURE 8.9: SEPARATING AND REFINING MEDITATION A #5 – BREATHE IN

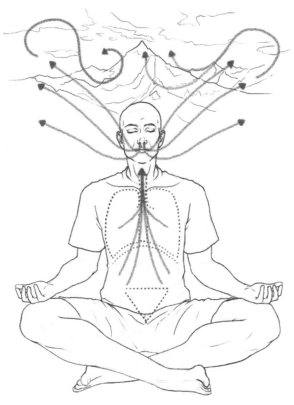

FIGURE 8.10: SEPARATING AND REFINING MEDITATION A #5 – BREATHE OUT

Separating and Refining Meditation B

1. Allow your breathing to settle, stop noticing it (perhaps by taking your attention somewhere else, like your back), and let it find its own rhythm.

2. Now take your attention to wherever you perceive your centre today. Take your time to feel exactly where that is, anatomically. Breathe in, and as you breathe out focus there again. Repeat several times. By breathing in and then focusing on this place as you exhale, you will start to have the sensation that you are breathing in and out from there, as if your lungs are located in that place.

3. Next time you breathe in, imagine that your breath is filling you up from your centre to the insides of your skin. The breath stretches your skin a little because of the internal expansion. If your centre is in your solar plexus, for example, just under your diaphragm, you might visualize the air filling your upper abdomen and expanding the skin at your sides, front and back so that you grow bigger, pushing against the elasticated insides of you. The air does not penetrate through the pores of your skin, it stays inside you, even if you get slightly bigger as you inhale. See Figure 8.11.

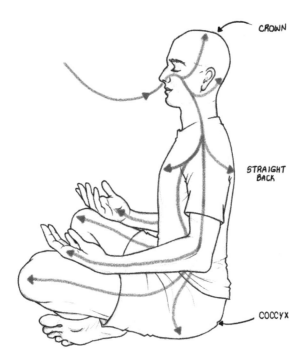

FIGURE 8.11: SEPARATING AND REFINING MEDITATION B #3 – BREATHE IN

4. Repeat this, experimenting with different body parts until you have a sense that all of you is one large organism (perhaps Masunaga's famous single-celled amoeba[2]) inhaling and exhaling, expanding and contracting as you breathe, keeping your breath

---

2   Masunaga's favourite vehicle for describing his theories was the one-celled animal, the amoeba (Beresford-Cooke 2011, p.147).

inside your own membrane, the dividing line between you and the rest of the world. Your breaths do not have to be long and it should not be a strain every time.

5. Keep breathing, and add an extra contraction on the exhalation: as you breathe out gently, tighten your anal sphincter. It is a light squeeze, like a reminder each time you breathe out to close a little extra in that region (that is, the end of the large intestine).

6. As this becomes easier, notice that you can still hear the noises around you, still smell the odours in the air, and feel where your hands touch your clothes as they rest on your lap or knees. Note that you can carry on with the breathing and squeezing and still be grounded, connected to the universe, contained and separate. Your breath, your Air Ki, reaches all the internal nooks and crannies of you, but it does not escape.

7. As it is getting towards the end of the meditation, allow your breathing to settle, and let it find its own rhythm. Stop noticing it and start a little smile.

8. To finish, once again lightly observe how you are – your body, feelings, thoughts and spiritual state. Do this mindfully so that you can compare with the scan you did earlier.

9. When you are ready, begin to move your fingers and toes, slowly nod or turn your head, reach forward with your hands along the floor, or the surface you are on, or out in front of you if you are on a chair, and stretch your fingertips in the opposite direction from your sitting bones. Pull your stomach muscles in towards your spine to curve your back and sit and then stand up.

You can make a recording of this and play it to yourself when you practise, until you know it. Use your best meditation voice. Alternatively, you can use the YouTube recording (Grainger 2019). Make notes in your self-development or continuing professional development journal about your experience or what you learned from the exercise afterwards.

The mantra is 'This is me' (see Figure 8.12).

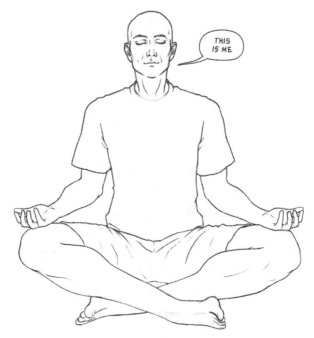

FIGURE 8.12: 'THIS IS ME'

The Lotus Blossom Opens Meditation

Aim: To develop acceptance and patience.

1. Sit or kneel, cross-legged or in seiza, with or without a chair, stool or cushion(s), finding a position and place which allows your spine to be straight – coccyx down to the earth and crown to the heavens, and your mind at peace. Rest your hands. Your eyes can be closed or open.

2. Lightly observe how you are today (that is, scan yourself), your feelings, thoughts and spiritual state, as if you are sitting in a beam of light which moves over and through you from top to toe collecting information or data about you in that instant. Do it lightly because it will not be useful in this context to attach any judgement to however you are, or make any changes to it unless they happen naturally and without effort, such as sitting up a bit straighter. Do all this mindfully so that you will have a residual memory of yourself for later comparison.

3. Notice your breathing: the air coming in and out of your nostrils, cool as it enters and warmer as it leaves. Listen to the sounds, observe the light and colours, and feel the quality of the air around you, smell the odours and taste the tastes you can detect. Be clearly aware, but decide not to be affected by them.

4. Mindfully move your hands up and join your palms in front of your Upper Burner (of the Triple Heater) where the heart and lungs are located. Press them very gently together. Almost imperceptibly move Chest Centre (Tanzhong Conception Vessel or Ren 17, Heart Governor/Heart Protector/Pericardium Bo or Mu point) and the sides of your thumbs towards each other. Pay attention to the place behind that acupressure point, in this moment, and then you will notice that you are breathing there.

5. Now let your hands gently move down to a comfortable place on your lap. Imagine a lotus flower bud growing where your breath is, behind Chest Centre (Tanzhong Conception Vessel or Ren 17, Heart Governor/Heart Protector/Pericardium Bo or Mu point); encased in smooth green leaves, its petals are hidden. Its roots are under the water, down in the mud (your Hara and pelvis, the Lower Burner), where it takes in nutrients and fluids. Page 167 of Veet Allan's *Ocean of Streams* (2006) shows a subsidiary branch of the Heart Governor (HG or Heart Constrictor/Heart Protector/Pericardium, HC/HP/P) which connects the oval-shaped diagnostic area with the pelvis like the roots of this energetic lotus flower. (This is in contrast to Masunaga's *Zen Shiatsu* (1977), which details the leg extensions crossing the fronts of the hips into the lower abdomen, but does not link it to the branch in the upper abdomen and chest.) The strong stalk, which connects the flower and the roots, rises up into the chest cavity. The Lower Burner is the lowest of the Three Burning Spaces/Triple Burner or Heater in TCM. Ted Kaptchuk (1983, p.69) quotes Qin Bo-wei *et al.* (1973) when he writes that 'The lower Burner is a swamp'.

6. As your breathing slows down, the flower expands and the dark green leaves begin to open, revealing the pale, delicate petals, its veins and subtle colours. In slow motion, it opens and you start to see the pink tips of the white flower, even its yellow centre.

You can smell the fragrance emanating from it. It is as if sunshine is coming out of the middle and warming your whole chest, as if you are shining from the inside outwards. Imagine that the nectar of your flower is there for insects to feast on, to collect and take away. If you are doing the meditation alone, for yourself, bask as long as you would like to. See Figure 8.13.

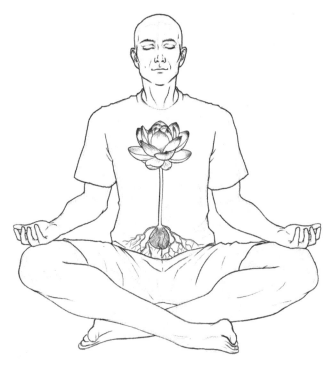

FIGURE 8.13: LOTUS FLOWER OPENING

7. If you are sitting beside your client doing this before a treatment, you can softly flutter your eyelids open and place one hand on their Hara and the other over their Chest Centre. The mantra is 'I am listening' (see Figure 8.14).

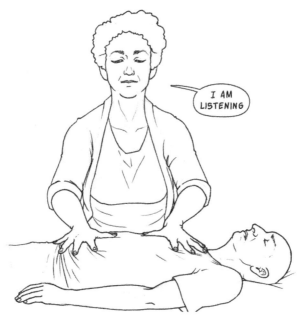

FIGURE 8.14: 'I AM LISTENING'

8. Then continue with the session. Say thank you and goodbye to your client as they leave. Then settle back down to carry out the following meditation conclusion. Do not forget this! Your heart is open for Shiatsu purposes and it will not serve you to be that open when you go back outside.

9. Meditation conclusion: Little by little, imagine it is the afternoon and your petals are starting to close as they naturally do when the light dwindles. Your eyes close. The nectar and all that warmth and sunlight is still inside, encased in the core. In your mind, as it gets darker towards night, the leaves also close and you rest quietly. Make a long exhalation to soften your chest. Take your palms over your closed eyes and feel the warmth through the lids bathing your eyeballs. When you are ready, open your eyes inside your hands and slowly open your fingers to let in the light. Bring your hands back to your lap or knees. Sit still for a while before stretching and getting up.

10. Now make notes in your self-development or continuing professional development journal about your experience or what you learned from the exercise.

Loving Kindness meditation

There is a well-known Buddhist practice for developing compassion called Metta Bhavana (the cultivation of loving kindness) from the Theravāda tradition. It is another very useful way to prepare yourself for this type of work. You are recommended to learn it from someone who can teach it well.

When you cannot tell someone something because they have died – a meditation

I came across this meditation so long ago that I cannot remember where it came from. It is for the unresolved issues: when you, the practitioner, or your client desperately wish you had said something before the person died ('sorry', 'goodbye', 'why?') and are finding it very hard to accept that you will never see them again to be able to do so. (I have also used it with someone who is still alive, but who I cannot or will not see again or with whom it is unsuitable to have such a conversation.) I have sometimes talked my clients through it, sitting with them as they are practising, and sometimes explained the exercise and left them to try it at home if they wanted.

Sitting quietly and comfortably, conjure up the person you want to talk to. Imagine she is above your head and see her there in as much detail as you can; then visualize sitting in front of her, looking into her eyes. Remember what it felt like to be with her, and sit there for a while. Choose your time, either say what you want to say – an apology, a reassurance or an expression of your anger or love – or have a conversation with her, allowing time for and hearing or sensing her replies. When you are finished, make sure you acknowledge that clearly and then say goodbye. Gently return to where you began, feeling the floor underneath you, your own body solid and breathing, and take time before opening your eyes.

You can be creative and adapt this to fit your own situation or your client's. Choose the time carefully, follow your instinct and, if you have any misgivings, do not use it.

Walking meditation

Walking meditation can teach patience and mindfulness. Being very slow and repetitive can help build up your leg muscles, and centre, ground and contain you. These are all skills which we need when we are working in extreme situations, on all four levels.

Decide where you want to do your walking meditation. Ideally you are alone in a beautiful place where you can walk barefoot without damaging your feet. Otherwise, choose somewhere inside. You require a place which is large enough not to have to turn corners every few steps as this takes more practice and awareness (and you might get giddy!). Having different floor coverings can be interesting as there are varying textures for you to walk onto and off again to bring your attention back to the ground when it wanders.

Sally Ibbotson (2019), Shiatsu practitioner and Qi gong teacher, reminds us: 'Part of the meditation in all qi gong is following your own rhythm of breathing…you follow your exhale, so only when you are empty of air is your foot fully weighted on the earth. I find this really important, so there is no hyperventilating and so that you are accepting yourself as you are.'

Option 1
It is very simple: Stand still in the Wu Chi stance as above (Figure 8.2). Breathe in and out deeply three times. Inhale as you step on the left foot, exhale as you step on the right, and so on.

Option 2
Alternatively, lift one foot slowly, peeling it away from the floor, balancing on the other foot and starting to fall forwards ever so slightly. At the beginning of the next inhalation the heel of that foot makes contact with the ground and the transfer of weight continues, and as your weight goes completely forwards onto the ball of that foot, exhale. Inhale as the heel of the other foot touches; exhale as your weight goes onto the ball of that foot. Repeat. The difference is that you breathe in and out on one foot rather than in on one and out on the other. This makes it slower and you have to balance more, using greater control.

Option 3
Do it with a partner. Choose which option above you are going to try and do it together. This teaches us to tune into someone else to enable

smooth movement and carry out a task together. The balance of power between one and the other, the decision to do what you want or to go with their rhythm, can be a delicate balance; the sense of togetherness in the task can be frustrating or supportive. All these aspects reflect the client–practitioner relationship and are tools for working with a client.

Reflection

How does this relate to working with clients at the end of life? How does doing this support you as the practitioner working with clients who have issues related to death and loss?

Here are some general reflection questions for practitioners:

- Have you nearly died or been given a life-threatening diagnosis? If so, how did you manage and what has changed as a result?

- Has someone you loved died? If so, how did you manage afterwards, and what has changed as a result?

- Do you notice that you ignore death or do you ever find yourself thinking that you could die at any time? What effect does this thinking or behaviour have on your life and Shiatsu?

- Do you approach death in the context of religion or in another spiritual context? If yes, what do you believe happens to you after you die?

- Are you scared of death?

- What sort of death do you want?

Start with a simple list of the ways you have engaged with death and loss to get you going. You may already have tried and tested ways that you use to engage with topics which inform your Shiatsu. If not, there are various ways you can start to look into your relationship with death and loss. Some ideas below tap into your subconscious, and others take a more methodical attitude:

- If you have a meditation practice or would like to start one, you can choose to use one of these questions as a focus. Choose one which attracts your attention and write it down or read it to yourself so that you remember it. While lighting a candle or sounding a bell, whatever you do to prepare for your sitting, hear the question in your head. Once settled, let it go and carry on as usual. Notice what arises.

- You can do the same with a walk, choosing one of these questions as a focus, writing it down or reading it as you prepare before you leave and then allowing your mind to quieten and make your perambulation, reflecting when you have finished.

- Journal writing, speaking into a microphone, drawing or doodling are other ways. Choose a question and write it at the top of a page. You can either put your pen or pencil down and sit quietly for a while before taking it up again and writing; alternatively, you can set a timer for some (five to ten) minutes, then place its tip on the page and write 'from your right brain', that is, let the words come out in a stream of consciousness – not judging them or stopping to reread, not worrying about making sentences or sense. When the timer sounds, you stop, have a stretch and then read what you have written and reflect on that.

- Consult the *I Ching*[3] or spread Tarot cards, using one of the questions.

- Write a letter to someone you love who has died but who was a great source of comfort when they were alive, telling them the question you are asking yourself.

- Choose a book which has inspirational writing in it – the *Tao De Ching*, Kahlil Gibran's *The Prophet*, Thich Nhat Hahn's *No Death, No Fear: Comforting Wisdom for Life*, a book of collected poetry by a writer you admire, or a book about death and dying you have obtained from the library. Choose your question from the list or make up your own, write it down and read it over a few times so that your Ki has heard and acknowledged it. Then hold the book between your two hands which are in the prayer position, shut your eyes and centre yourself, breathe in and out deeply three times with the question in your mind, and let the book fall open. Read the page(s) and see if anything you find there is illuminating.

---

3 'The Yijing (or "Book of Change") is…an oracle, yes, but also has a philosophy around it of…the life and death of all living things' (Bertschinger 2015).

- Take a large piece of paper and some coloured pens or pencils and write the question in the centre. Using the mind map technique of arrows and balloons, brainstorm on the subject, making your mind map as colourful as you like, until you have a poster to place on your wall. You can add to it as you walk past, or after breakfast, making extra lines to join the word clouds together if they seem to be linked, or colouring parts differently as you change your mind or have another thought.

- Use a spreadsheet to make a table with the numbered questions in the left-hand column and your answers in the right. Update it as necessary.

- Visit a place which has a spiritual significance for you – a beach, a clearing in the woods or the top of a hill perhaps. Choose your question and, as you make your way there, collect things which draw your attention – leaves, stones, sticks, flowers. When you arrive, arrange them in a way which pleases you, while having the question in your mind. When you have finished, stand back, dedicate it to someone who has died, maybe take a photo, and leave it in nature's hands.

- In a town or city, visit a church and sit quietly, or go to a cemetery and take a wander around – with the question in your mind.

— Chapter 9 —

Conclusion

Working with people who are facing death and loss is a privilege. End-of-life care brings us into contact with our priorities, tests our strength, shows us how we manage suffering and focuses on our degree of attachment to the world and the people in it. It brings us into contact with our relationship to the spiritual dimension in a way no other work does. Death is levelling, something all life on earth shares, and if we are open to learning and exchanging the true spirit of Shiatsu, there is no reason why we cannot develop into more highly evolved beings. Yes, the Yin and Yang of Ki means that we are doing this serious and vital work at a time when our natural world, and therefore everything else, is threatened by the effects of pollution, greed and zest for power over others. However, we are lucky: our work reminds us, on a daily basis, that there is kindness in the world alongside the suffering; it gives us tools for building up resilience and finding peaceable ways to counter conflict.

The longer I stay with Shiatsu, the more I feel that the practice and underlying theory offer us a way to deal with all aspects of life, should we choose to use it. In the context of this book, it is the intimate touch of Shiatsu allied with the careful and respectful use of words; the acutely observed way we diagnose the client's gestures and posture; the practitioner's own approach informed by a deep energy practice and heightened awareness, that are ideal for the types of encounters which involve loss and death.

Chapter 2 of this book examined the way that Ki, Yin and Yang, the Five Phases, TCM and Zen and Quantum Shiatsu pertain to its topics. It imagined, or told of, clients in scenarios on all four levels and applied our philosophy to them. Whether working in a generally instinctive way using protocols sparingly, or using diagnosis and specific techniques, the aim was that you would find the theory pertaining to the dying and grieving processes interesting and valuable in your work. Perhaps you have a greater understanding of your grieving client's Ki, or the patterns of symptoms your end-of-life client is exhibiting now, and I would like to think that you are more confident with what you know, and aware of the safety considerations, including understanding how to assess when Shiatsu is appropriate or not.

As well as identifying who dies of what in the UK, USA and Australia, and where, Chapters 3 and 4 addressed the various ways our clients live, die or respond to death and grief. They went into the possible causes of suicide and the way other cultures and religions have historically managed and currently deal with the end of life and the mourning period. Throughout, there were real case studies to bring the theory to life.

Chapter 5 looked at the practitioner, tackling the thorny issue of how to talk about death, and the practical steps to take in preparation for our own demise and how to support our clients through that. Self-care and supervision, working alongside other professionals and embodying professionalism, plus working with family and friends, were examined. I hope you will be uninhibited in accessing support when you need it in the future. This chapter included some extreme situations where fellow practitioners are undertaking valuable humanitarian work, and it contained a discussion about remaining compassionate in the face of our own threatened death, or that of a loved one, while maintaining our practice. I hope you will remember to REST – to REflect, have Supervision and get some Therapy (which of course really meant enjoy a Shiatsu!) in order to stay balanced and open in this powerful work.

The client–practitioner relationship was the subject matter of Chapter 6, looking at how we engage with what goes on between us, spoken and unspoken, some of which is comparable to the work of our counselling colleagues, particularly of issues which arise when suffering is paramount. It looked at the essence of communication, of power between us, at managing expectations and pressure, maintaining boundaries, at listening and, above all, at love.

Managing death in the teaching environment, both as a topic on the curriculum and when it affects the student body or tutor itself, was the focus of Chapter 7. In the spirit of continuing professional development and co-education, there were exercises and discussion topics for practitioners to share.

Finally, Chapter 8 offered meditations and Qi gong for building strength and protection. Additionally, there were other ways to stimulate and reflect on the way death has affected us, to prepare ourselves for this thought-provoking work, for the stillness and clear limits required.

In one way, working with people who are grieving or at the end of life is the same as giving Shiatsu to anyone: whatever they are going through can be seen as a shift of Ki, and we therefore treat them as special individuals who need care. In another way, it is useful, less nerve-racking, and much safer to be informed in advance about the manner in which our health institutions are run and how we fit in with their teams; to begin to know what impact death has had on us personally; and to be aware of the types of behaviour our clients may exhibit when facing these stages of life.

As to the Shiatsu techniques, well, you will notice that I have not often told you what to do or how to touch someone who is grieving or dying, although I have made suggestions. This is because of the myriad varieties of situations you will find yourself in and the wonderful individuality of each person we touch. As soon as I encourage you to use the Lung meridian with someone who is sad, you will meet a client who needs grounding, so that she can sort out her own ways to cope, and so the Kidney meridian will be called for to promote rest and relaxation. I could say that anyone who is on their deathbed requires a spiritual approach, and then you would meet someone who has bed sores and will not be able to concentrate on anything else until they get some relief. As with all our clients, there is no one person the same as any other. So, the absolute best we can do is prepare assiduously, inform ourselves with care, and focus on self-support so that we are as healthy and resilient as our lives allow and can therefore offer our loving touch in a manner which is safe for us all.

At the dawn of every day, in the face of our constant nearness to death, I advise you to – as Steven Levine (1997, p.20) exhorts – 'practise living'.

Shiatsu is...

Shiatsu is a Japanese touch therapy. It is suitable and appropriate to be offered to patients as complementary to conventional medical practice, and Shiatsu practitioners must complete a rigorous three-year training, including anatomy, physiology and pathology. It can support patients who are undergoing the diagnosis and challenges of medical treatment and its side effects and needing relaxation in the face of stress. It can help with symptom control, including nausea, pain management and improved mobility, and increase energy levels to enable people to remain active where possible up until the point of death (as per NHS aims). It can also improve emotional resilience with clarity of thought when patients are feeling vulnerable and uncertain around death and dying. In the case of relatives and carers of the dying, the combined listening skills and care through touch supports the grieving process.

Shiatsu practitioners are able to:

- offer verbal alongside touch therapy to ascertain needs

- address physical, emotional, mental and spiritual issues concurrently

- give recommendations and suggest exercises

- teach self-Shiatsu to patients

- teach relatives to give Shiatsu to patients

- understand the medical diagnosis and operate safely with it

- work closely and in an informed way with physiotherapists, occupational therapists, chaplaincy, counsellors, doctors and nurses, as well as other specialists

- support patients through conventional treatment.

Shiatsu is referred to patients who may be either in a care setting because they are dying, attending someone's death, or suffering complications of grief and loss.

Comparing the Western and Eastern Models, and Comparing Complementary to Alternative Medicine

Comparing the Western and Eastern models

There are a range of differences between the Shiatsu (generally, Eastern) and the Western medical approaches to clients/patients and their treatment.

The use of pharmacologically active agents or physical interventions by Western medical staff to treat or suppress symptoms or pathophysiologic processes of diseases or conditions with cases of cancer and other serious diseases as well as at the end of life can be immeasurably useful, especially acute ones, for the short term, or with dogged and life-interrupting situations, thereby saving lives. The consultants, physicians, nursing staff and ambulance workers, plus all the ancillary staff, are highly trained; however, it is unlikely that they will have much time available to spend with each patient or with us if we work alongside them, and they may well be dealing with many people at one time.

If we can be the ones who are there to give the patient a hug or say a kind word, then we are filling a gap and that is an example of the complementary aspect that we are aiming for. By no means is this all we offer, but neither should we underestimate that. Patients appreciate such treatment, resulting in positive feedback, and the hospital and charity employers lay great store by this. The early aim of medicine (Young 1871) was 'the preservation and improvement of health', and more recently has been stated, 'to save and prolong life, fight and prevent diseases, reduce pain and sufferings' (Jakusovaite and Darulis 2004). The latter pertains to death and loss – bringing patients back from coma, for example, keeping them alive as long as possible, and administering medications at the end of life. Patients can now sign an Advance Decision to Refuse Treatment (ADRT) or make a Living Will including the refusal for life-sustaining or life-saving treatments (National Health Service 2017). In contrast, our practice is to promote health and self-healing in the circumstances the client requests, including at the end of life. If they state that they are ready to die, or want to prepare themselves emotionally or spiritually as well as mentally and physically to die, we will support them. We aim to provide time and space for the client to find a way to express what they are feeling and indicate what they are looking for, and the hospital staff will be using tried and tested, general rather than individualized procedures.

If we are working with a familiar client who has been admitted to hospital or to the hospice, we know their Ki, how they behaved beforehand. Instinctively, we know where they are on the life/end-of-life scale of the bodymind. Not all Shiatsu practitioners understand the biological aetiology or course or natural history of the disease as accurately as the medical staff do.

What might be uncomfortable for us in any hospital situation, particularly if we are present over a prolonged period of time, is that the treatment and procedures used are fundamentally different from our Shiatsu ways. We are so familiar with a mind-body-spirit attitude that the clinical, one-body-system-at-a-time approach may be hard to accept. In Chinese Medicine, we look for the pattern of symptoms; we consult our own Ki; we are alert to the Ki in the field; we are looking for a relational diagnosis which addresses the four levels of physical, emotional, mental and spiritual; and we use all of our faculties: visual, aural, smell and taste, as well as touch. Traditional medical staff will also verbally question to ascertain and test hypotheses, and use machines to measure and 'see' with the aim of finding a fit with one of their possible scenarios. The procedures and medications used in medical centres are tried and tested by science. Please refer to Table B.1: The differences between Eastern and Western medicine.

Table B.1: The differences between Eastern and Western medicine

Western	Eastern
Dualistic – mind/body split	Holistic – treats whole person
The medical personnel are focused on and specialists in the patient's pathology	The patient knows best The whole person is the focus
Diagnosis using scientific cause/effect	Diagnosis looks at patterns
Concerned with eradicating germs and pathogens	Starts with health, wellbeing and balance in life
Effective with acute illness and symptom management	Effective with chronic illness and symptom management
Uses medication and surgery	Non-invasive, no medication used
Training focused on treatment of disease	Training focused equally on treatment and practitioner attitude
Applicable when disease or illness is present	Preventative care and treatment
Part of the government or private healthcare systems	Generally independent
Recognized by government and scientists	Voluntarily registered

Complementary or alternative medicine

Most Shiatsu practitioners prefer to be part of *complementary* rather than *alternative* therapies. Many Shiatsu practitioners aim to become integrated with mainstream medical services so that patients and clients can access a full range of support for wellbeing and health, chronic and acute issues including auto-immune and mental health issues. Governments across the English-speaking world are struggling to provide effective healthcare options for everyone, particularly those who are unable to fund their own. The current health services are very expensive and the number of people requiring them is growing. We have so much to offer in this medical context and our aim is to co-exist harmoniously with them.

— Appendix C —

Research

In the *Shiatsu Society (UK) Journal*, Mercedes Núñez (2013, p.12) writes: 'We often bemoan the fact that not enough research is being done to show how effective our therapy is. But, working with cancer has shown me that medical research *already* validates Shiatsu practice. This should give us tremendous confidence to continue doing what we do.'

There are no major scientific research programmes looking at the use of Shiatsu in the areas of grief, loss or palliative care, but there are a few minor studies. 'Explaining the value of Shiatsu in palliative care day services' (Cheeseman, Christian and Cresswell 2001) is a qualitative one, reported in the *International Journal of Palliative Nursing* (US), which revealed significant improvements in patient energy levels, relaxation, confidence, symptom control, clarity of thought and mobility which were of variable duration, from a few hours to extending beyond the five-week treatment. Another US study conducted by a nurse who is also a Shiatsu practitioner has suggested that Shiatsu may assist with grief, pain management, nausea and insomnia (Stevenson 1995).

The most in-depth, longitudinal cohort research into Shiatsu was presented in 2007 by Professor Long at the University of Leeds and looked at who receives Shiatsu (Spain, Austria and the UK), why people choose to engage with it, client–practitioner interaction, effectiveness in the longer term, safety and negative factors, and the economic benefits. Research methodologies, such as double-blind trials, are inappropriate for Shiatsu, so this was a qualitative study.

A notable, though small study looked at the impact on a GP surgery of having a complementary therapist as part of the team in Sheffield, England (Pirie 2003).

Innovative research is currently being carried out into energy medicine, particularly by Patrizia Stefanini (a Shiatsu practitioner and quantum physicist) in Italy and by James Oschman (author of *Energy Medicine: The Scientific Basis* (2015)) in the US.

The British Acupuncture Council (Standish, Kozak and Congdon 2008) states, 'Of 27 RCTs on acupuncture for conditions seen frequently in palliative care, 23 reported statistically significant, favourable results.' The authors concluded that acupuncture is safe and clinically cost-effective for the management of common symptoms in palliative and end-of-life care.

There has been some research into Tai Chi, looking at symptoms, with a growing body of evidence that people sustain a range of significant health benefits (for improved balance, arthritic pain relief, cardio-vascular health and a decrease in the numbers of pro-inflammatory lymphocytes circulating) as a result (Deadman n.d.).

The Research Council for Complementary Medicine (CAM)[1] and the National End-of-Life Intelligence Network (Gov.UK Collection 2019) both have interesting information to offer on research into complementary and alternative medicine and end-of-life care respectively.

There is a good report on the *Taking Charge of Your Health and Wellbeing* website by Pamela Miles and Deborah Ringdahl (2016) about research and Reiki which is applicable to Shiatsu, though not specifically about death and loss.

In her PhD study Zoe Pirie (2003, p.2) notes:

> The existing literature states that '...the popularity of complementary therapies is growing rapidly' (Vincent and Furnham, 1998) with 30% of the British public being treated by complementary practitioners every year (Sharma, 1992) and 75% claiming that it should be made available on the National Health Service (MORI Poll, 1989). Recent governmental policies that introduced primary care groups in 1999 and encouraged the further research of complementary medicine (House of Lords report, 2000) are helping to make this a reality with 40% of general practices now offering access to complementary medicine (Zollman and Vickers, 1990). However, there is little research on how to integrate complementary medicine into general practice (Robinson and Berman, 1984).

---

1   Research Council for Complementary Medicine Evidence and Best Practice: www. rccm.org

See also the article by Robinson, Lorenc and Liao (2011), which provides a systematic review of Shiatsu and acupressure, the Shiatsu Society (UK) website[2] and the European Shiatsu Federation.[3]

2   www.shiatsusociety.org/shiatsu-research
3   www.europeanshiatsufederation.eu/en/research

Glossary

Beginner's mind: from Buddhism. An attitude of possibility without preconceptions.

Bereavement: the experience of having lost someone who you cared for.

Blood, Essence/Jing, Shen: three of the Vital Substances of TCM.

Bodymind: holistic terminology. Used in this book to denote the whole person including the physical, emotional, mental and spiritual aspects of the human being.

Clean Language: 'Clean Language is a set of questions that help the client to explore and transform their own subjective reality with minimum interference from the questioner' (Pole 2017, p.27). Developed by David Grove.

Cremation: a service or ceremony during which a body is burned, usually held in the chapel of the crematorium.

End-of-life care: care for the elderly and others who are at the final stage of life. Carried out as above for palliative care (see Chapter 4).

Expressions of the Zen Meridian pairs: Metal: to yawn (and stretch); Earth: to grasp something to eat; Water: to flee; Wood: to turn from side to side; Primary Fire (HT and SI): to contemplate, to pray; Secondary Fire (HG and TH): to hug oneself or protect from the cold.

Funeral: a service or ceremony during which a body is buried. Traditionally held on 'hallowed ground' in a church but increasingly taking place elsewhere.

Grief: the response to the loss of someone or something. Can be physical, emotional, mental or spiritual.

Hara: the centre, located in the abdominal region.

Ki/Chi/Qi: Ki is the Japanese form of the Chinese word Qi or Chi, for which there is no satisfactory translation. In Chinese, the word contains the radicals for both 'steam' and 'rice', indicating something both insubstantial and physically palpable, a subtle energy which can condense into substance. Ki is the basis of all phenomena, whether something you can or cannot hold onto, whether animate or inanimate, concrete or in the realm of feeling. Ki is commonly referred to as 'energy' in English, which, as it has the Yang properties of warming, transforming and activating, means that we can use the Newtonian physics definition: 'the ability to do work'. Importantly, given the subject of this book, when Ki is not present, the physical system is not animated. It is said that if there is no longer movement of Ki, the organism is dead. (With thanks to Carola Beresford-Cooke.)

Kyo and Jitsu: Zen Shiatsu terminology, a relationship between two (akin to Yin Yang) often described as feeling empty and full, or hidden and obvious, respectively.

Loss: the absence of someone or something. Also a synonym for death.

Memorial: an opportunity to celebrate the life of the one who has died. Can be distinct from the funeral or wake, for the general public or extended friends and colleagues of the deceased, and can take place up to a year after death. Suitable in cases where there is no body to bury.

Meridian: perceived energy channel through which Ki travels.

Mother and active hands: the still, listening and accepting hand; and the other hand which moves from place to place, making stationary contact as well as receiving information. They are intrinsically connected.

Mourning: a period of mourning is the time allocated to remembering and showing others that this is happening. It is also a term for the clothes worn by those who are grieving.

Near or nearing death awareness: not the same as each other: near death awareness commonly refers to the experience of those who nearly die, but are resuscitated; nearing death awareness denotes experiences some have before death and can involve talking to those who have already died, and speaking about or preparing for what will happen next.

Off-body Shiatsu: (related to Light Body) Shiatsu without touching the physical body.

Organ: of Zang Fu, often taking the name of the physical organ, but denoting an action throughout the bodymind.

Palliative care: care for those who are seriously or terminally ill. Can be offered at home, in hospital, hospice or other residential setting. Consists of allopathic and complementary treatment, psychotherapy, chaplaincy, art and music (see Chapter 4).

Po (Corporeal Soul which exists when the body has breath – Metal element), **Hun** (Ethereal Soul which exists after the death of the body – Wood element), **Shen** (Awareness – Fire element), **Zhi** (Will – Water element), **Yi** (Intellect, thoughts – Earth element): the Five Shen (spiritual capacities) of TCM (see Chapter 2).

Scattering of ashes: the dissemination of the ashes created at the cremation, often in nature or a place holding important memories for the deceased or their family.

Stages of the life-cycle of the amoeba: 1) LU/LI: making a border and initiating exchange; 2) SP/ST: satisfying needs; 3) HT/SI: assimilating and integrating nourishment; 4) KD/BL: flight from danger; 5) HG/TH: circulation and protection; 6) LV/GB: choice of direction (Beresford-Cooke 2011, pp.153–157).

Tao: often translated as way (guidance to being in the world). Defies definition. From Taoism (Chinese) – see *Tao Te Ching*.

TCM: Traditional Chinese Medicine.

The Five Elements/Phases: Metal, Earth, Fire, Water and Wood from TCM (see Chapter 2).

Tsubo: Japanese word meaning 'vase'. An acupressure point found along a meridian.

Wake: the presentation of someone in their opened coffin. Can be in a domestic setting, chapel or care home. Can be for family only or the public. It is also the name given to the party or gathering for refreshments held after a funeral.

Yin Yang: 'In Taoist cosmology, Yin and Yang are the two archetypal principles produced by the movement and stillness of the Void… and by their interaction they together create Ki and the world of phenomena' (Beresford-Cooke 2011, p.117). Mutually arising and interdependent, all four principles of Yin and Yang which are written about in more detail in Chapter 2 tell us something about death and loss.

Zen Meridian functions according to Masunaga: Lung and Large Intestine: breathing and excretion; Spleen and Stomach: obtaining food and digestion; Heart and Small Intestine: central control and conversion; Bladder and Kidney: purify and give impetus; Triple Heater and Heart Constrictor (Protector): circulation and protection; Liver and Gallbladder: stocking and distribution (Beresford-Cooke 2011, Fig. 11.6, p.152).

Zen/Movement/Quantum/Seiki/Barefoot Shiatsu: styles or modes of Shiatsu (see Chapter 2).

Meridian or channel abbreviations

BL: Bladder

CV: Conception Vessel, also Ren Mai, one of the central channels

GB: Gallbladder

GV: Governing Vessel, also Du Mai, one of the central channels

HG/P/HP: Heart Governor/Pericardium/Heart Protector

HT: Heart

KD: Kidney

LI: Large Intestine

LU: Lung

LV: Liver

PV: Penetrating Vessel, also Chong Mai, one of the Extraordinary Vessels

SI: Small Intestine

SP: Spleen Pancreas

ST: Stomach

Tai Yin: one of the Six Stages or Divisions (Lung and Spleen meridians)

TH: Triple Heater

Further Reading and Resources

Government policy

Definition of Palliative Care (2019) World Health Organization. www.who.int/cancer/palliative/definition/en.

End of Life Care Strategy (England, UK) (2008) Department of Health. https://assets.publishing.service.gov.uk/government/uploads/system/uploads/attachment_data/file/136431/End_of_life_strategy.pdf.

Health and Social Care Delivery Plan Health and Social Care (2016) Healthcare Quality and Improvement Directorate (Edinburgh, Scotland). www.gov.scot/publications/health-social-care-delivery-plan/pages/2.

Recommendation Rec (2003) 24 of the Committee of Ministers to member states on the organization of palliative care (2003) Council of Europe. www.coe.int/t/dg3/health/Source/Rec(2003)24_en.pdf.

Seymour, J. and Cassel, B. (2016) 'Palliative care in the USA and England: a critical analysis of meaning and implementation towards a public health approach.' *Mortality* 22 (4) 275–290.

General

Boerstler, R. and Cornfield, H. (1995) *Life to Death: Harmonizing the Transition.* Rochester, VT: Healing Arts Press.

Bush, M. and Dass, R. (2018) *Walking Each Other Home, Conversations on Loving and Dying.* Louisville, CO: Sounds True Publishing.

Byock, I. (1998) *Dying Well.* New York, NY: Riverhead Books.

Callanan, M. and Kelley, P. (1992) *Final Gifts: Understanding and Helping the Dying.* London: Hodder and Stoughton.

Chopra, D. (2006) *Life After Death: The Book of Answers* (includes physics and Vedic info as well as Buddhist). New York, NY: Random House.

Didion, J. (2005) *The Year of Magical Thinking.* New York, NY: Alfred A. Knopf.

Gawande, A. (2014) *Being Mortal.* New York, NY: Metropolitan Books.

Goswami, A. (2001) *Physics of the Soul: The Quantum Book of Living, Dying, Reincarnation and Immortality.* Charlottesville, VA: Hampton Roads Publishing Company.

Halifax, J. (2008) *Being with Dying: Cultivating Compassion and Fearlessness in the Presence of Death*. Boston, MA: Shambhala.

Holloway, R. (2018) *Waiting for the Last Bus*. Edinburgh: Canongate Books.

Kübler-Ross, E. and Kessler, D. (2005) *On Grief and Grieving*. New York, NY: Simon and Schuster.

Lief, J.L. (2001) *Making Friends with Death*. Boston, MA: Shambhala Publications.

Lind-Kyle, P. (2017) *Embracing the End of Life: A Journey into Dying and Awakening*. Woodbury, MN: Llewellyn Publications.

Levine, S. (1984) *Meetings at the Edge: Dialogues with the Grieving and the Dying, the Healing and the Healed*. New York, NY: Anchor Press.

Levine, S. (2017) *Healing into Life and Death*. England and New York, NY: Anchor Press/Doubleday.

Mannix, K. (2017) *With the End in Mind: Dying, Death and Wisdom in an Age of Denial*. New York, NY: William (Harper) Collins.

Marsh, H. (2014) *Do No Harm*. London: Weidenfeld and Nicolson.

McCartney, M. (2014) *Living with Dying*. London: Pinter and Martin.

Modi, S. (2014) *In Love with Death*. Edinburgh: Birlinn.

Nepo, M. (2012) *Seven Thousand Ways to Listen: Staying Close to What is Sacred*. London: Simon and Schuster.

Nuland, S.B. (1994) *How We Die: Reflections on Life's Final Chapter*. New York, NY: Alfred A. Knopf.

Rinpoche, S. (1992) *The Tibetan Book of Living and Dying*. London: HarperCollins.

Wanzer, S. and Glenmullen, J. (2007) *To Die Well: Your Right to Comfort, Calm and Choice in the Last Days of Life*. Cambridge, MA: Da Capo Lifelong Books.

Whyte, D. (1990) *Where Many Rivers Meet*. Langley, WA: Many Rivers Press.

Wilbur, K. (1991) *Grace and Grit*. Boston, MA: Shambhala Publications.

After death

Boerstler, R. and Cornfield, H. (1995) *Life to Death: Harmonizing the Transition*. Rochester, VT: Healing Arts Press.

Roach, M. (2003) *Stiff: The Curious Lives of Human Cadavers*. New York, NY: WW Norton.

Japan's traditions

Onishin, N. (2018) *Why Japan's Ageing Population is Dying Alone*. Available at www.scmp.com/magazines/post-magazine/long-reads/article/2139153/lonely-deaths-why-japans-ageing-population-dying.

For the dying

Albom, M. (1997) *Tuesdays with Morrie*. New York, NY: Doubleday.

Green, J. (2013) *The Fault in Our Stars*. London: Penguin.

Kuhl, D. (2002) *What Dying People Want: Practical Wisdom for the End of Life*. Cambridge, MA: Perseus Books.

Near death experiences

Alexander, E. (2012) *Proof of Heaven*. New York, NY: Simon and Schuster.

Alexander, E. and Tompkins, P. (2014) *The Map of Heaven: How Science, Religion, and Ordinary People Are Proving the Afterlife*. New York, NY: Simon and Schuster.

Fitzpatrick, R. (2015) *Taking Heaven Lightly: A Near Death Experience Survivor's Story and Inspirational Guide to Living in the Light*. Dublin, Ireland: Hachette Books.

Kean, L. (2017) *Surviving Death: A Journalist Investigates Evidence for an Afterlife*. New York, NY: Crown Archetype.

Keane, C. (2009) *Going Home: Irish Stories from the Edge of Death*. Dungarvan, Co. Waterford, Ireland: Capel Island Press.

Keane, C. (2014) *Heading for the Light: The 10 Things That Happen When You Die*. Dungarvan, Co. Waterford, Ireland: Capel Island Press.

Historical

Kelly, J. and Lyons, M.A. (eds) *Death and Dying in Ireland, Britain and Europe: Historical Perspectives*. Sallins, Co. Kildare, Ireland: Irish Academic Press.

Grief

Devine, M. (2017) *It's OK That You're Not OK: Meeting Grief and Loss in a Culture That Doesn't Understand*. Louisville, CO: Sounds True Publishing.

James, J.W. and Friedman, R. (2001) *When Children Grieve*. New York, NY: HarperCollins.

James, J.W. and Friedman, R. (2009) *The Grief Recovery Handbook*. New York, NY: HarperCollins.

Jozefowski, J. (1999) *The Phoenix Phenomenon: Rising from the Ashes of Grief*. Northvale, NJ: Jason Aronson.

Morris, S. (2012) *Overcoming Grief*. London: Constable and Robinson.

Samuel, J. (2017) *Grief Works: Stories of Life, Death and Surviving*. London: Penguin Life.

Wright, J. (2014) *Back to Life*. https://www.recover-from-grief.com/support-files/back-to-life.pdf.

Loss

Coleman, P. (2014) *Finding Peace When Your Heart is in Pieces*. London: Adams Media.

The Loss Foundation, charity: www.thelossfoundation.org.

Death/End-of-life doula

Fersko-Weiss, H. (2017) *Caring for the Dying: The Doula Approach to a Meaningful Death*. Newburyport, MA: Conari Press.

Hebb, M. (2018) *Let's Talk About Death (over Dinner)*. Boston, MA: Da Capo Lifelong Books.

Herring, L. (2019) *Reimagining Death: Stories and Practical Wisdom for Home Funerals and Green Burials*. Berkeley, CA: North Atlantic Books.

Okun, B. and Nowinski, J. (2011) *Saying Goodbye: How Families Can Find Renewal Through Loss*. New York, NY: Berkeley Publishing.

Volandes, A.E. (2015) *The Conversation: A Revolutionary Plan for End-of-Life Care*. New York, NY: Bloomsbury.

Find more titles like these at: www.goodreads.com/shelf/show/death-doula.

Other

Doughty, C. (2015) *Smoke Gets in Your Eyes – A Mortician's Dissection of Death*. Available at www.theguardian.com/books/2015/may/03/smoke-gets-in-your-eyes-review-caitlin-doughty-and-other-lessons-from-the-crematorium.

Edge, S. (2018) *Don't Wait, Celebrate Yourself*. YouTube, Goalcast.

Hsieh, J-G. and Wang, Y-W. (2012) 'Application of signs of dying identified in traditional Chinese, Tibetan, and modern Western medicine in terminal care.' *Tzu Chi Medical Journal* 24:1, 12–15. Available at www.sciencedirect.com/science/article/pii/S1016319012000067.

Hughes, K. (2014) *The Journey into Spirit: A Pagan's Perspective on Death, Dying & Bereavement*. Woodbury, MN: Llewellyn Publications.

Koudounaris, P. (2011) *The Empire of Death: A Cultural History of Ossuaries and Charnel Houses*. London: Thames and Hudson.

Magnusson, M. (2017) *The Swedish Art of Death Cleaning: How to Free Yourself and Your Family from a Lifetime of Clutter*. London: Canongate Books.

Mendoza, M.A. (2018) *Professional Mourners: An Ancient Tradition*. Available at www.psychologytoday.com/us/blog/understanding-grief/201802/professional-mourners-ancient-tradition.

Mitford, J. (1963, revised 1996) *The American Way of Death*. New York, NY: Simon and Schuster.

Muslim/Islamic traditions: https://cremationinstitute.com/muslim-funeral-traditions.

Patrick Caulfield's Grave featured in Darkest London blog: https://darkestlondon.com/2011/05/04/patrick-caulfields-grave-in-highgate.

Peters, D., Chaitow, L., Harris, G. and Morrison, S. (2001) *Integrating Complementary Therapies in Primary Care: A Practical Guide for Health Professionals*. Amsterdam: Elsevier.

Pole, N. (2018) *Words that Touch: How to Ask Questions Your Body Can Answer – 12 Essential 'Clean Questions' for Mind/Body Therapists*. London: Singing Dragon.

Schillace, B. (2017) *Death's Summer Coat: What the History of Death and Dying Teaches Us About Life and Living*. New York, NY: Pegasus.

The Departure Lounge – research-led public event in Lewisham, London. With Academy of Medical Sciences: https://acmedsci.ac.uk and www.theguardian.com/lifeandstyle/2019/may/05/welcome-to-the-deaprture-lounge-destination-death.

Wailing: https://en.wikipedia.org/wiki/Death_wail.

Shiatsu Society Journal articles

Henderson-Haefner, D. (2017) 'Working with the dying' (141) 15–16.

Stefanini, P. (2000) 'Quantum physics and Shiatsu' (72) 2–4.

Stefanini, P. (2001) 'Masunaga in quantumland' (75) 24–25.

Websites

Annetta Black (Odd Salon, Time Travel Project and Death Salon co-organizer), San Francisco: https://annettablack.com. Interview with her here detailing all sorts of death stories, a talk she gave on Dr Benjamin Lyford and his new embalming methods which allowed him to send dead soldiers back to their families, and the beginnings of her book: https://lorenrhoads.com/2014/10/09/death-salon-interview-annetta-black.

Contemplation on death, meditation: https://integrallife.com/contemplation-on-death-impermanence.

Death Cafe: https://deathcafe.com.

Death Salon – mortality and mourning through the lenses of art, history and culture: https://deathsalon.org (Los Angeles, London, San Francisco)

Holding space: https://heatherplett.com/2015/03/hold-space.

Lucretius (2015, 1st century BC) *De Rerum Natura (On the Nature of the Universe)*, Book 3. See Stanford Encyclopedia of Philosophy Section 4. Physics, Book 3.

Memento Mori Collective: https://challenges.openideo.com/challenge/end-of-life/research/the-memento-mori-society.

The 7 Stages of Grief: www.recover-from-grief.com/7-stages-of-grief.html.

The Art of Dying Well (Catholic): www.artofdyingwell.org.

The Death Project: https://susanbriscoe.wordpress.com/recommended-reading-2.

The Good Grief Project: https://thegoodgriefproject.co.uk.

The Sinking Ship, Death, Dying and Chinese Medicine: www.windhorsemedicine.com/musings/sinking-ship-death-dying-chinese-medicine.

Yin Yang House – acupuncture website for location and names of acupressure points: https://yinyanghouse.com.

Museums and galleries

Barts (St Batholomew's Hospital, London) Pathology Museum, Queen Mary University of London: www.qmul.ac.uk/pathologymuseum. Holds events related to death and dying from a pathology point of view, for example 'Facing Death': Death Masks (with Nick Reynolds of Memorial Casts) in 2018, and the UK Death Salon Conference in 2014.

Dangerous Perfection: Funerary Vases from Southern Italy. J.P. Getty Museum, Los Angeles (2015): www.getty.edu/art/exhibitions/apulian_vases.

Personal books/articles about someone in the family dying

Bowler, K. (2018) *Everything Happens for a Reason (and Other Lies I've Loved)*. London: SPCK Publishing.

Coutts, M. (2014) *The Iceberg*. London: Atlantic Books.

Didion, J. (2005) *The Year of Magical Thinking*. New York, NY: Alfred A. Knopf.

Didion, J. (2011) *Blue Nights*. New York, NY: Alfred A. Knopf.

Hitchens, C. (2012) *Mortality*. London: Atlantic Books.

Kalanithi, P. (2016) *When Breath Becomes Air*. New York, NY: Random House.

Lourde, A. (1980) *The Cancer Journals*. San Francisco, CA: Aunt Lute Books.

Pausch, R. (2008) *The Last Lecture*. Sydney, Australia: Hachette Books.

Rapp, E. (2013) *The Still Point of the Turning World*. New York, NY: Penguin.

Riggs, N. (2017) *The Bright Hour*. Waterville, ME: Thorndike Press.

Robinson, J.G. (2017) 'Road to recovery.' *New York Times*. Available at www.nytimes.com/2017/12/07/travel/road-trip-family-grief.html?_r=0&module=inline.

Sacks, O. (2015) *Gratitude*. New York, NY: Alfred A. Knopf.

Scott, R. (2019) *Between Living and Dying: Reflections from the Edge of Experience*. Edinburgh: Birlinn.

Taylor, C. (2017) *Dying: A Memoir*. Portland, OR: Tin House Books.

Chronic illness

Bailey, E.T. (2010) *The Sound of a Wild Snail Eating*. Cambridge: Green Books.

Poetry

Darling, J. (2003) *Sudden Collapses in Public Places*. Available at http://juliadarling.co.uk/works/poetry/sudden-collapses-in-public-places.

Heaney, S. (1975) 'Funeral Rites'. In *North*. London: Faber.

Larkin, P. (2012) 'Aubade'. In A. Burnett (ed.) *The Complete Poems*, pp.115–116. London: Faber and Faber.

Novels

Mansell, A. (2018) *I Wanted to Tell You: An Emotional and Heartbreaking Story about Love and Loss*. London: Bookouture.

Philosophy and death

Critchley, S. (2008) *On Heidegger's Being and Time*. Abingdon, Oxfordshire: Routledge.

Heidegger, M. (1967) *Being and Time*. Oxford: Blackwell.

Lacewing, M. (n.d.) Aristotle, the Soul and Life After Death. Available at www.alevelphilosophy.co.uk/handouts_religion/AristotleSoulLifeAfterDeath.pdf.

Blogs and articles

Avery, H. (n.d.) *Serving the Dying: End of Life Doulas*: https://wanderlust.com/journal/serving-the-dying-end-of-life-doulas.

Bloom, W. (2017) *Death – Facilitating the Transfer of Consciousness*: https://williambloom.com/2017/01/24/death-facilitating-the-transfer-of-consciousness.

Confessions of a Funeral Director: www.calebwilde.com.

Diary of a Widower: https://diaryofawidower.com.

Grief Healing Blog: www.griefhealingblog.com.

Heidegger's Being and Time: https://philosophyblognssr.wordpress.com/classes/spring-2015/heideggers-being-and-time-simon-critchley.

Hello Grief: www.hellogrief.org.

Rose, J. (2014) *10 Bittersweet Things You Learn when You Lose Someone You Love*: https://thoughtcatalog.com/jessica-rose/2014/07/10-bittersweet-things-you-learn-when-you-lose-someone-you-love/?fbclid=IwAR0TDJ05D17_TWz7Ad5Zd3m2l83pxfE8_rzJK3Gn_-h9zzN-1AuXs9KV3lY.

Still Standing Magazine: https://stillstandingmag.com/2016/06/01/welcome-to-still-standing-magazine.

Wilfried Rappanecker's articles on Zen Shiatsu, and on pain by others: www.schule-fuer-shiatsu.de/shiatsu/veroeffentlichungen/englische-artikel.html.

Training

Being With Dying, set up by Joan Halifax: www.upaya.org/being-with-dying.
Scottish Compassionate Communities Toolkit: www.goodlifedeathgrief.org.
uk/content/toolkit_homepage.

Death doula training

Doulagivers. Certified end-of-life training: www.doulagivers.com.
Quality of Life Care. *Accompanying the Dying: A Practical Guide and Awareness Training*. https://www.qualityoflifecare.com/uploads/3/4/0/3/3403119/end_of_life_doula_training_-_2019_brochure.pdf.
Tucker, E. (2014) *What on Earth is a Death Cafe?* www.theguardian.com/lifeandstyle/2014/mar/22/death-cafe-talk-about-dying.

Videos

Ask a Mortician, All My Fave Graves, Iconic Corpse and more on YouTube with www.youtube.com/user/OrderoftheGoodDeath.
Documentary about The Silent Teacher – a medical school where they call the cadavers their 'silent teacher' and treat the body and the family with respect: https://vimeo.com/190986528?fbclid=IwAR3I2nzvhLjF4wkvNVnrtZopnKB89hrxf9_7Mdqr0Rf5PdYUADbpk3agL1I.
Gaia has videos such *as Dying to Wake Up* and *The Fun of Dying*: www.gaia.com.
Grief Actually: https://vimeo.com/286865132?ref=fb-share&1.
To Absent Friends: www.toabsentfriends.org.uk/content/about-film.
Under the Knife (Dr Lindsey Fitzharris). This episode is about The Death House – 'the grim reality facing medical students in earlier centuries when they first entered the dissection room, or "dead house," as they called it'. Also check out Al Capone and syphilis: www.youtube.com/watch?v=AuKG0NOZvnk.

Films

Frankel, D. (director) (2016) *Collateral Beauty*.
Itami, J. (director) (1984) *The Funeral*.
Takita, Y. (director) (2008) *Departures*.
Unkrich, L. (director) (2017) *Coco*.

Radio

Why Grief Is Not Something You Have to Get Over (2018) BBC Sounds.

TV shows

Ball, A. (2001) *Six Feet Under*: www.imdb.com/title/tt0248654. In addition, one of the characters is a Shiatsu practitioner.

BBC Ideas playlist on death and dying: www.bbc.com/ideas/playlists/dying-thoughts.

Gervais, R. (2019) *After Life*. Netflix: www.imdb.com/title/tt8398600.

Golaszewski, S. (2016) *Mum*. iPlayer.

Events

Death cafe. Set up in the UK by the late Jon Underwood to create the non-profit Death Cafe in 2011, based on the Swiss Cafe Mortel movement: https://deathcafe.com.

Dying to Know Day: 8/8/2019, Australia.

The Sisters of Doom and Gloom, an event held in 2019 for Death Awareness Week. Check to see if there are more events: www.facebook.com/events/moncrieff-church/the-sisters-of-doom-and-gloom-lets-talk-about-death/1620002354809343.

References

Abramović, M. (2013) Accessed 31.8.19 at www.youtube.com/watch?v= BwPTKmFcYAQ.

Agular, G. (2015) 'Shiatsu in the hospice wards, "A felt journey".' *Shiatsu Society UK Journal,* Issue 133, 10.

Alexander, P. (1951) Hamlet (Shakespeare, W.) *The Alexander Text of the Complete Works of Shakespeare.* London and Glasgow: Collins.

Allan, V. (2006, originally published in 1994) *Ocean of Streams: Zen Shiatsu, Meridians, Tsubos and Theoretical Impressions.* Thornhall: Omki.

Almeida, G. (2019) *Portugal Declares Day of Mourning for Domestic Violence.* Reuters. Accessed 30.8.19 at www.reuters.com/article/us-portugal-government-domesticviolence/portugal-declares-day-of-mourning-for-domestic-violence-victims-idUSKCN1QH2BV.

American Psychiatric Association (2013) *Diagnostic and Statistical Manual of Mental Disorders: DSM-5* (fifth edition). Arlington, VA: American Psychiatric Publishing.

Andrews, C. (2004) 'Treating joints with Shiatsu.' *Shiatsu Society UK Journal,* Issue 91, 11.

Andrews, C. (2012) *Kyo and Jitsu: An Evolving Part of Shiatsu Energy Work.* Accessed 09.03.20 at https://www.europeanshiatsucongress.eu/wp-content/uploads/2016/11/1611-ARTIKEL-CLIFF-ANDREWS-KYO-AND-JITSU.pdf.

Andrews, C. (2018) 'Treating stress and trauma.' *Shiatsu Society UK Journal,* Issue 148, 14.

Andrews, C. (2019) *New Energy Work.* Accessed 27.8.19 at www.newenergywork.com.

Arundel, L. (2019) In conversation with the author.

Bailey, T. (1999) *A Better Approach to Complementary Therapy.* Positive Health Online. Accessed 31.8.19 at www.positivehealth.com/article/bodywork/a-better-approach-to-complementary-therapy.

BBC (2019) *Bitesize: Life after Death.* Accessed 31.8.19 at www.bbc.com/bitesize/guides/zhxpr82/revision/3.

BBC News (2019) *Scotland has Highest Drug Death Rate in EU.* Accessed 31.8.19 at www.bbc.co.uk/news/uk-scotland-48938509.

Beinfeld, H. and Korngold, E. (1992) *Between Heaven and Earth: A Guide to Chinese Medicine.* New York, NY: Ballantine Books (Random House). From the introduction.

Beresford-Cooke, C. (2011) *Shiatsu Theory and Practice* (third edition). Edinburgh: Elsevier.

Berry, W. (2012) 'The Peace of Wild Things'. In *New Collected Poems.* Berkeley, CA: Counterpoint Press.

Bertschinger, R. (2015) 'Yijing. Have all of Chinese Medicine in your pocket – interview'. Blog: Singing Dragon. Accessed at http://singingdragon.com/sdblog/tag/yijing.

Callanan, M. and Kelley, A. (2012) *Final Gifts: Understanding the Special Awareness, Needs and Communications of the Dying.* New York, NY: Simon and Schuster.

Cancer Research UK (2019) *Cancer Mortality Statistics.* Accessed 1.7.19 at www.cancerresearchuk.org/health-professional/cancer-statistics/mortality.

Castellino, Dr R. (2000) 'The Stress Matrix: Implications for Prenatal and Birth Therapy' *Castellino, Prenatal and Birth Therapy Training.* Accessed 09/03/2020 at http://www.castellinotraining.com/products.

Chan, C.L.W. and Chow, A.Y.M. (2006) 'Introduction, Chinese Culture and Death.' In C.L.W. Chan and A.Y.M. Chow (eds) *Death, Dying and Bereavement: A Hong Kong Chinese Experience.* Hong Kong: Hong Kong University Press.

Cheeseman, C., Christian, R. and Cresswell, J. (2001) 'Explaining the value of Shiatsu in palliative care day services.' *International Journal of Palliative Nursing* 7 (5) 234–239.

Churcher, S.J., from Facebook group, *Everything Shiatsu* thread, with permission.

Complementary and Natural Healthcare Council (UK) (2018) *Code of Conduct, Ethics and Performance.* Accessed 30.9.19 at www.cnhc.org.uk/sites/default/files/Downloads/CodeofConductEthicsandPerformance.pdf.

Crisis Centre (2013) *Frequently Asked Questions.* Canada. Accessed 30.9.19 at https://crisiscentre.bc.ca/frequently-asked-questions-about-suicide.

Cystic Fibrosis Foundation (2017) *Patient Registry Highlights.* Bethesda, MD: Cystic Fibrosis Foundation.

Day of the Dead (Dia de los Muertos) (2018) Accessed 31.8.19 at www.history.com/topics/halloween/day-of-the-dead.

Deadman, P. (n.d.) *Qigong and Tai Chi Research.* Accessed 28.8.19 at https://peterdeadman.co.uk/qigong/qigong-and-tai-chi-research.

Devine, M. (n.d.) *How Do You Help a Grieving Friend?* Refuge in Grief. Accessed 27.8.19 at www.refugeingrief.com.

Dr Dan Keown (n.d.) https://m.youtube.com/watch?v=XnDG8L_nXhw& feature=youtu.be. See also *The Spark in the Machine* and *The Uncharted Body*.

Draper, E., Gallimore, I., Kurinczuk, J., Smith, P. *et al.* (2018) *MBRRACE-UK Perinatal Mortality Surveillance Report: UK Perinatal Deaths for Births from January to December 2016*. Available at www.npeu.ox.ac.uk/downloads/files/mbrrace-uk/reports/MBRRACE-UK%20Perinatal%20Surveillance%20Full%20Report%20for%202016%20-%20June%202018.pdf.

Duquesne School of Nursing (n.d.) *Roles and Responsibilities of a Community Healthcare Nurse*. Accessed 25.8.19 at https://onlinenursing.duq.edu/blog/roles-responsibilities-community-health-nurse.

eCondolence.com (US) (n.d.) *Understanding Shinto: Japanese Tradition and Ritual Provide Comfort for Mourners*. Accessed 31.8.19 at www.econdolence.com/learn/articles/shinto-understanding-shinto.

Engel, C. (2018) 'Somatic empathy in Shiatsu: the science (pt 1).' *Shiatsu Society UK Journal*, Winter issue, 148.

Fairweather, R. and Mari, M.S. (2019) *Jing Advanced Massage Training*. Accessed 27.8.19 at www.jingmassage.com.

Federal Insurance Contributions Act Tax. Wikipedia (2019) Accessed 27.8.19 at https://en.wikipedia.org/wiki/Federal_Insurance_Contributions_Act_tax.

Fennell, J. (2019) In conversation with the author.

Fischer, K. (2018) *How 'Death Doulas' Can Help People at the End of Their Life*. Healthline. Accessed 27.8.19 at www.healthline.com/health-news/how-death-doulas-can-help-people-at-the-end-of-their-life#1.

Funeral Guide (2017) *Colours of Mourning Around the World*. Accessed 31.8.19 at www.funeralzone.com.au/blog/mourning-colours.

Gaertner-Webster, M. (2019) Personal communication.

Gardoni, A. (2018) '*Very, Very Traumatic' Working with Trauma using Clean Language and Shiatsu by Nick Pole MRSS(T) and Peter Cadney*. Accessed 1.9.19 at www.shiatsualiceg.co.uk/very-very-traumatic-working-with-trauma-using-clean-language-and-shiatsu-by-nick-pole-mrsstand-peter-cadney.

Gov.UK Collection (2019) *Palliative and End of Life Care*. Accessed 2.1.20 at www.gov.uk/government/collections/palliative-and-end-of-life-care.

Grainger, T. (2019) *Separating and Refining Meditation*. Tamsin Grainger on YouTube.

Granek, L. (2012) *When Doctors Grieve*. The New York Times Sunday review. Accessed 31.8.19 at www.nytimes.com/2012/05/27/opinion/sunday/when-doctors-grieve.html?mtrref=www.google.co.uk&gwh=4B65DB58A71DD03E5B718FAC9CFEA25B&gwt=pay&assetType=REGIWALL.

Greene, J. (2019) *Once More We Saw Stars.* London: Hodder and Stoughton.

Groombridge, J. (2019) In conversation with the author.

Haelle, T. (2018) *Doctors and the D Word: Talking About Death is an Essential Skill and One Often Lacking.* Medical Bag. Accessed 25.8.19 at www.medicalbag.com/home/medicine/doctors-and-the-d-word-talking-about-death-is-an-essential-skill-and-one-often-lacking.

Hall, K. (Summer 2010) 'Shiatsu in psychiatric care.' *Shiatsu Society UK Journal,* Issue 114, 6–8.

Hansen, V. (2000) *The Open Empire: A History of China to 1800.* London: WW Norton and Company.

Healthcare Quality and Improvement Directorate (2016) *Health and Social Care Delivery Plan.* Edinburgh. Accessed at 31.8.19 at www.gov.scot/publications/health-social-care-delivery-plan/pages/2.

Helbert, K. (2019) *The Chakras in Grief and Trauma.* London: Singing Dragon.

Holder, B. (2018) *Poverty Link to Early Death 'Scandalous'.* BBC News. Accessed 30.8.19 at www.bbc.co.uk/news/uk-england-44853482.

Hospitals Contribution Fund of Australia (HCF) (2019) *Health Expectancy: How Long Can You Live?* Accessed 11.12.19 at www.hcf.com.au/health-agenda/health-care/research-and-insights/life-expectancy-in-australia.

Ibbotson, S. (2019) *Qigong: Fragrant Buddha.* YouTube: accessed 11.12.19 at https://youtu.be/qxTcm0fZSYk.

Itin, P. (2009) 'Shiatsu for the consequences of trauma.' *Shiatsu Society UK Journal,* Issues 110 and 111.

Jaggs, F. (2019) In conversation with the author.

Jakusovaite, I. and Darulis, Z. (2004) 'Values and goals of medicine and healthcare.' US National Library of Medicine, National Institutes of Health US. Accessed 30.8.19 at www.ncbi.nlm.nih.gov/pubmed/15456967.

Jenkins, K. (2017) *Year 2 Worksheet* (with permission).

Jenkins, K. (2019) In conversation with the author.

Johnson, A.J. (2002) 'Energetic anatomy and physiology.' *Chinese Medical QiGong Therapy,* Vol. 1, 120.

Jong, J., Ross, R., Philip, T., Chang, Si-H. *et al.* (2017) 'The religious correlates of death anxiety: A systematic review and meta analysis.' *Religion, Brain, & Behaviour,* Vol. 8, Issue 1, www.tandfonline.com/doi/abs/10.1080/2153599X.2016.1238844?journalCode=rrbb20.

Kaptchuk, T.J. (1983) *Chinese Medicine: The Web that has No Weaver.* London: Rider (Random House).

Kishi, A. and Whieldon, A. (2011) *Life in Resonance: The Secret Art of Shiatsu.* London: Singing Dragon.

Kübler-Ross, E. (2019, originally published 1959) *On Death & Dying: What the Dying Have to Teach Nurses, Doctors, the Clergy and their Own Families.* Scribner, kindle edition.

Kübler-Ross, E. and Kessler, D. (2005) *On Grief and Grieving*. New York, NY: Simon and Schuster.

Langford, D. (2014) A Truly Victorian Experience. *The Etiquette of Mourning*. Tinker Swiss Cottage Museum, UK.

Lao Tzu (trans. U. Le Guin, with the collaboration of J.P. Seaton) (2011) *Tao Te Ching: A Book about the Way and the Power of the Way*. Boston and London: Shambhala Publications.

Larkin, P. (2012) Aubade. In A. Burnett (ed.) *The Complete Poems*, pp.115–116. London: Faber and Faber.

Leadbeater, C.W. (2007, first published 1912) *A Textbook of Theosophy*. New York, NY: Cosimo Classics UK.

Learning Disability Today (2016) *Largest English Study into Health and Care of People with Learning Disabilities Published Today*. NHS Digital.

Lee, M.C., Hinderer, K.A. and Alexander, C.S. (2018) *What Matters Most at the End-of-Life for Chinese Americans?* US National Library of Medicine National Institutes of Health. Available at www.ncbi.nlm.nih.gov/pmc/articles/PMC6050625.

Levine, S. (1997) *A Year to Live*. New York, NY: Three Rivers Press.

Loeb, A. (writer), Frankel, D. (director) (2016) *Collateral Beauty*.

Long, A.F. (2007) *The Effects and Experience of Shiatsu: A Cross-European Study. Final Report*. Accessed 28.8.19 at http://eprints.whiterose.ac.uk/42957.

Love, D. (2019) *Life Options*. Death Doula Australia. Accessed 31.8.19 at www.deathdoulaaustralia.com.

Lu, W., Doherty-Gilman, A.M. and Rosenthal, D.S. (2010) 'Recent advances in oncology acupuncture and safety considerations in practice.' *Current Treatment Options in Oncology* 11(3–4) 141–146.

Lucretius (trans. W.E. Ellery; intro. C. Bailey) (2015) *De Rerum Natura: Of the Nature of Things*. New York, NY: Walter J. Black. For Classics Club.

Maciocia, G. (1989) *The Foundations of Chinese Medicine*. Edinburgh: Churchill Livingstone.

MacLeod, R.D., Wilson, D.M. and Malpass, P. (2012) 'Assisted or hastened death: the healthcare practitioner's dilemma.' *Global Journal of Health Science* 4(6) 87–96.

Macmillan Cancer Support (2017) *Macmillan Nurses*. Available at www.macmillan.org.uk/information-and-support/coping/getting-support/macmillan-nurses.html.

Mannix, K. (2017) *With the End in Mind: Dying, Death and Wisdom in an Age of Denial*. New York, NY: William (Harper) Collins.

Marie Curie (n.d.) *What to Expect from Our Nurses*. Accessed 25.8.19 at www.mariecurie.org.uk/help/nursing-services/what-marie-curie-nurses-do/what-to-expect-from-our-nurses.

Masunaga, S., with Ohashi, W. (1977) *Zen Shiatsu: How to Harmonize Yin and Yang for Better Health*. Tokyo and New York, NY: Japan Publications.

Mead, S. (n.d.) (founder) Intentional Peer Support. *What is IPS?* Accessed 27.8.19 at www.intentionalpeersupport.org/what-is-ips.

Medicine Net Newsletter (2018) *The Medical Version of Hippocratic Oath.* Accessed 27.8.19 at www.medicinenet.com/script/main/art.asp?articlekey=20909.

Miles, P. and Ringdahl, D. (2016) *What Does the Research Say About Reiki? Taking Charge of Your Health & Wellbeing.* University of Minnesota. Accessed 1.9.19 at www.takingcharge.csh.umn.edu/explore-healing-practices/reiki/what-does-research-say-about-reiki.

Monroe, M.H. (2010) *Australia, The Land Where Time Began: Death and the Afterlife.* Accessed 31.8.19 at https://austhrutime.com/aboriginal_death_afterlife.htm; and *The Afterlife: The Aboriginal Australian Afterlife.* Accessed 31.8.19 at http://lifeafterdeathinformation.weebly.com/aboriginal-afterlife-beliefs.html.

Mulholland, B. (2012) *Touching the End of Life: Shiatsu and Death.* Shiatsu Year 3 Dissertation.

Murray Parkes, C., Laungani, P., Young, B. and Young, W. (2015) *Death and Bereavement Across Cultures.* Oxford: Routledge.

My Jewish Learning (n.d.) *The Basics of Kriah, or Tearing a Piece of Clothing.* Accessed 31.8.19 at www.myjewishlearning.com/article/the-basics-of-kriah-or-tearing-a-piece-of-clothing.

National Cancer Institute (2018) USA. *Cancer Statistics.* Accessed 1.7.19 at www.cancer.gov/about-cancer/understanding/statistics.

National Health Service (2017) *Advance Decision (Living Will).* Accessed 29.9.19 at www.nhs.uk/conditions/end-of-life-care/advance-decision-to-refuse-treatment.

National Health Service (2019) *Maternity and Neo-natal Services.* Accessed 25.8.19 at www.longtermplan.nhs.uk/online-version/chapter-3-further-progress-on-care-quality-and-outcomes/a-strong-start-in-life-for-children-and-young-people/maternity-and-neonatal-services.

National Health Service (2019) *Stillbirth.* Accessed 1.9.19 at www.nhs.uk/conditions/stillbirth.

National Health Service Scotland (2006) *A Multi-Faith Resource for Healthcare Staff.* Accessed 6.1.20 at www.nes.scot.nhs.uk/media/3720/march07finalversions.pdf.pdf.

National Institute of Mental Health US (2017) *Suicide.* Accessed 1.9.19 at www.nimh.nih.gov/health/statistics/suicide.shtml.

National Institute of Mental Health US (2019, report of 2017 figures) *Major Depression.* Accessed 31.8.19 at www.nimh.nih.gov/health/statistics/major-depression.shtml.

National Institute on Aging US (2017) *What Are Palliative Care and Hospice Care?* Accessed 29.9.19 at www.nia.nih.gov/health/what-are-palliative-care-and-hospice-care.

National Records of Scotland (2017) *Vital Events Reference Tables 2017*. Accessed 6.1.20 at www.nrscotland.gov.uk/statistics-and-data/statistics/ statistics-by-theme/vital-events/general-publications/vital-events-reference-tables/2017.

Nelissen, T. (2005) 'Hara Shiatsu in clinical institutions.' *Shiatsu Society UK Journal*, Issue 93, 3.

Nhat Hanh, T. (2002) *No Death, No Fear: Comforting Wisdom for Life.* London: Ebury/Rider.

NHS Health Research Authority and Medical Research Council (2019) *Consent and Participant Information Guidance*, version 7. Accessed 13.12.19 at www.hra-decisiontools.org.uk/consent/principles-deceased.html.

Nordqvist, C. (2018) Reviewed by Legg, T.J. Medical News Today. *What are Euthanasia and Assisted Suicide?* Healthline Media UK.

Núñez, M. (2013) 'Cancer medicine.' *Shiatsu Society UK Journal*, Issue 127.

Nursing Times (n.d.) *District Nursing.* Accessed 25.8.19 at www.nursingtimes. net/district-nursing/5004050.article.

O'Brien, S.B. (2017) *Doulagivers.* Accessed 25.8.19 at www.doulagivers.com.

O'Hagen, S. (2017) *My Father's Wake by Kevin Toolis. Review – A Brutal Epiphany.* Available at www.theguardian.com/books/2017/aug/29/my-fathers-wake-kevin-toolis-review-a-brutal-epiphany-irish-teach-us-to-live-love-and-die.

Office for National Statistics (2017) *Causes of Death over 100 Years.* Accessed 31.8.19 at www.ons.gov.uk/peoplepopulationandcommunity/ birthsdeathsandmarriages/deaths/articles/causesofdeathover100years/ 2017-09-18.

Office for National Statistics (2018a) *National Life Tables, UK 2015–2017.* London: ONS.

Office for National Statistics (2018b) *Deaths Registered in England and Wales (series DR) 2017.* London: ONS. Accessed 1.7.19 at www.ons.gov. uk/peoplepopulationandcommunity/birthsdeathsandmarriages/deaths/ bulletins/deathsregisteredinenglandandwalesseriesdr/2017.

Oschman, J.L. (2015) *Energy Medicine: The Scientific Basis* (second edition). Edinburgh: Elsevier.

Palmer, B. (1996) 'The Six Divisions.' *Journal of Shiatsu and Oriental Body Therapy*, Issue 5. Accessed 30.9.19 at www.seed.org/articles/sixdivisions. pdf.

Palmer, B. (2011) 'Working with elders.' *Shiatsu Society UK Journal*, issue 120.

Palmer, B. (2013) *Tiger in the Grove: Kyo and Jitsu in Movement.* Accessed 30.9.19 at www.seed.org/articles/tiger_in_grove.pdf.

Palmer, B. (2019) Personal correspondence.

Personal and Professional Development: What is Mentoring? University of Cambridge, UK. Accessed 27.8.19 at www.ppd.admin.cam.ac.uk/professional-development/mentoring-university-cambridge/what-mentoring.

Pirie, Z. (2003) *The Impact of Delivering Shiatsu in General Practice.* Available at https://core.ac.uk/download/pdf/20343880.pdf.

Pole, N. (2017) *Words that Touch: How to Ask Questions Your Body Can Answer.* London: Singing Dragon.

Pooley, N. (2000) 'The meridians: Lung and Large Intestine.' *Shiatsu Society UK Journal,* Issue 73, 12.

Pooley, N. (2001) 'The different vibrational levels of the meridians.' *Shiatsu Society UK Journal,* Issue 79, 21.

Qin Bowei *et al.* (1973) *Traditional Chinese Medical References for Clinical Patterns (Zhong-yi Liong-chuan Bei-yao).* Beijing: People's Press.

Rappenecker, W. (2001) 'Shiatsu with Heart Energy.' *Shiatsu Society UK Journal,* Issue 80, 2.

Rappenecker, W. (2017) *Energetic Perception.* Austria: European Shiatsu Congress workshop.

Reoch, R. (2000, first published 1997) *Dying Well: A Holistic Guide for the Dying and Their Carers.* London: Gaia Books Ltd.

Robinson, N., Lorenc, A. and Liao, X. (2011) 'The evidence for Shiatsu: a systematic review of Shiatsu and acupressure.' *BMC Complementary and Alternative Medicine,* article number 88. Accessed 1.9.19 at https://bmccomplementalternmed.biomedcentral.com/articles/10.1186/1472-6882-11-88.

Rochat de la Vallee, E. and Larre, C. (1995) *Rooted in Spirit: The Heart of Chinese Medicine.* New York, NY: Station Hill Press.

Rules of Sport.com (n.d.) *What is the World's Most Dangerous Sport?* Accessed 31.8.19 at www.rulesofsport.com/faq/what-is-the-world-s-most-dangerous-sport.html.

Rumi. *Out Beyond Ideas.* National Poetry Day (Forward Arts Foundation) (n.d.) Accessed 13.12.19 at https://nationalpoetryday.co.uk/poem/out-beyond-ideas.

Sanchez, D. (2001) 'Shiatsu in the aftermath.' *Shiatsu Society News,* Winter, number 80.

Sasaki, P. (2001) *The Evolution of Shiatsu.* Transcript of the online seminar hosted by Pauline Sasaki and Cliff Andrews, New Energy Work, pdf 6/23.

Scotland NHS Lothian (2019) *Palliative Care.* Accessed 30.9.19 at https://services.nhslothian.scot/palliativecare/Pages/default.aspx.

Sheldon, L. (2019) In private correspondence.

Sheppard, G. (n.d.) *The Issue of Confidentiality When a Client Dies.* Canadian Counselling and Psychotherapy Association. Accessed 27.8.19 at www.ccpa-accp.ca/wp-content/uploads/2015/05/NOE.Issue-of-confidentiality-when-a-client-dies.pdf.

Shiatsu Society (UK) (n.d.) *Code of Conduct and Ethics*. Accessed 27.8.19 at https://ssuk-public-test.aptsolutions.net/media/78/78.pdf.

Shuford, C. (2019) *Zen Shiatsu*. Accessed 09.03.20 at https://www.carol zenshiatsu.com.

Shuken, C. (2013) 'Taking up the Slack.' Workshop handout. Edinburgh.

Singh, G. (2019) *Sikhism and Ageing*. Sikh Missionary Society. Accessed 27.8.19 at www.sikhmissionarysociety.org/sms/smsarticles/advisorypanel/gurmukhsinghsewauk/sikhismandageing.

Sipper, J. (n.d.) *The Tibetan Book of the Dead: Summary, Translation & Quotes*. Study.com. Accessed 27.8.19 at https://study.com/academy/lesson/the-tibetan-book-of-the-dead-summary-translation-quotes.html.

Sravasti Abbey (n.d.) *A Day in the Life*. Accessed 27.8.19 at https://sravastiabbey.org/who-we-are/day-in-lif.

Staib, A. (2019) Personal communication.

Standish, L.J., Kozak, L. and Congdon, S. (2008) 'Acupuncture is underutilized in hospice and palliative medicine.' *American Journal of Hospice and Palliative Care*. Aug–Sept; 25(4) 298–308.

Stevenson, C. (1995) 'The role of Shiatsu in palliative care.' *Complementary Therapy in Nursing and Midwifery* 1(2) 51–58.

Strapps, A. and Hunter, J. (2017) *Shiatsu Workforce Australia*. Shiatsu Therapy Association of Australia. Accessed 27.8.19 at www.staa.org.au/resources/Documents/Workforce%20survey%20Pt%201.pdf.

Superguide (2019) *Understanding Your Life Expectancy*. Australian Bureau of Statistics (2017) Accessed 1.7.19 at www.superguide.com.au/boost-your-superannuation/latest-data-find-out-how-long-you-can-expect-to-live.

Tadhg Jonathan (2018) *Surrounded by a Great Cloud of Witnesses…Thoughts about Samhain*. Accessed 27.8.19 at https://tadhgtalks.me.

Terzani, T. (2004) *One More Ride on the Merry-Go-Round*. Uttar Pradesh, India: HarperCollins India.

Time to Change (2019) *Violence & Mental Health*. Accessed 27.8.19 at www.time-to-change.org.uk/media-centre/responsible-reporting/violence-mental-health-problems.

T-Knox (2019) *Colors of Mourning*. Accessed 09.03.20 at https://www.funeralguide.net/blog/mourning-colours.

Today on YouTube (2018) *What is it Like to Survive a Suicide Attempt?* Accessed 31.8.19 at www.youtube.com/watch?v=BW_FcyqQPb4.

Twicken, D. (2004a) 'Taoist models of Hun and Po, Part One.' *Acupuncture Today*, Volume 5, issue 8.

Twicken, D. (2004b) 'Taoist models of Hun and Po, Part Two.' *Acupuncture Today*, Volume 5, issue 9. Accessed 6.1.20 at www.acupuncturetoday.com/mpacms/at/article.php?id=28537.

Underwood, J. (2011) *Death Cafe*. Accessed 31.8.19 at https://deathcafe.com.

United Nations. Department of Economic and Social Affairs, Disability (n.d.) *Article 9 – Accessibility*. Accessed 25.8.19 at www.un.org/development/desa/disabilities/convention-on-the-rights-of-persons-with-disabilities/article-9-accessibility.html.

Victoria State Government, Australia, (2018) *Mental Illness and Violence*. Accessed 31.8.19 at www.betterhealth.vic.gov.au/health/ConditionsAndTreatments/mental-illness-and-violence.

Westwood, C. (2019) In conversation with the author.

Whieldon, A. (2018) *Seiki Shiatsu and Mindclearing*. Available at https://living-in-resonance.com/sei-ki-workshops.

Whiting, R. (2019) In conversation with the author (email). Refugee Advocacy, Information and Support, Lancaster. Accessed 1.9.19 at http://rais.org.uk.

Wikipedia (2019a) *Elysium*. Accessed 31.8.19 at https://en.wikipedia.org/wiki/Elysium.

Wikipedia (2019b) *Japanese Funeral*. Accessed 31.8.19 at https://en.m.wikipedia.org/wiki/Japanese_funeral.

Wikipedia (2019c) *The Summerland*. Accessed 31.8.19 at https://en.wikipedia.org/wiki/The_Summerland.

Women's Aid Federation of England (2015) *Domestic Abuse and Your Mental Health*. Accessed 31.8.19 at www.womensaid.org.uk/the-survivors-handbook/domestic-abuse-and-your-mental-health.

World Health Organization (1980) *A Manual of Classification Relating to the Consequences of Disease*. Geneva: International Classification of Impairments, Disabilities and Handicaps.

World Health Organization (2002) *National Cancer Control Programmes: Policies and Managerial Guidelines*. Geneva: WHO.

World Health Organization (2019a) *Definition of Palliative Care*. Accessed 1.9.19 at www.who.int/cancer/palliative/definition/en.

World Health Organization (2019b) *Tobacco*. Accessed 31.8.19 at www.who.int/news-room/fact-sheets/detail/tobacco.

Yates, S. (1990) *Wellmother*. Accessed 1.9.19 at www.wellmother.org.

Yates, S. (2018) *The Body Keeps Score*. Accessed 1.9.19 at www.wellmother.org/body-keeps-score.

Yeats, W.B. (n.d.) *The Cold Heaven*. Accessed 1.9.19 at www.poetryfoundation.org/poems/43287/the-cold-heaven.

Young, J. (1871) 'The aims of medicine.' *British Medical Journal*. Accessed 1.9.19 at www.bmj.com/content/1/543/553.

Yu, A.C. (1987) 'Rest, rest, perturbed spirit!: ghosts in traditional Chinese prose fiction.' *Harvard Journal of Asiatic Studies* 47(2) 403.

Subject Index

clients *cont.*
venues for meeting 112–20
wish for death of child 141 *see also*
client-practitioner relationship
co-counselling 196
Code of Conduct and Ethics (Shiatsu
Society) 160, 209–10, 218, 224
*Code of Conduct, Ethics and
Performance (CNHC)* 210
contraindications 78
Corporeal Soul *see* Po
crown chakra 74
cultural practices of clients
burial rituals 169–73
dedications 175
funeral ceremonies 167–8
ideas of afterlife 164–6
mourning 166–7
spirits 175–9
storytelling 173–4
wakes 168–9
cycle of life 29–32

death
acceptance of another 144–5
attending 127–9, 131–2
beliefs about 35
causes of 111–12
in cycle of life 29–32
death doulas 131–2
definition of 29
fear of 28–9, 151–2
and Five Elements 52–65
of infants 87–90, 134–5
journey into 15–17
and Ki 39–40, 41
metaphors for 32
place of 124–6
of practitioner 207–13
practitioners facing 181–6
signs of 129–31
and Traditional Chinese
Medicine 42, 47–8
vocabulary for 27–8, 32–4
death doulas 131–2
death threats 225–6
depression 153–5
diagnosis difficulties 75–6

*Diagnostic and Statistical Manual
of Mental Disorders (DSM-5)*
(American Psychiatric
Association) 153
disability 133–4
*Dying Well - A Holistic Guide for the
Dying and Their Carers* (Reoch) 21

Earth
connection to death 57–8
embarrassment 84–5
end-of-life Shiatsu 200–3
euthanasia 163–4
exercises
Gathering of Essence and Shen 281–4
guided meditations 285–98
Lotus Blossom Opens
meditation 292–5
Loving Kindness meditation 296
Qi gong 273–8
reflections on 298–300
separating and refining
meditations 286–91
Standing Like a Tree 274–9
walking meditation 296–8
expectations in client-practitioner
relationship 237–8

faith of clients 133
burial rituals 169–73
dedications 175
funeral ceremonies 167–8
ideas of afterlife 164–6
mourning 166–7
spirits 175–9
storytelling 173–4
wakes 168–9
fear of death 28–9, 151–2
feedback from clients 79–80
Fire
connection to death 58–9
Five Elements
connection to death 52–4
and Earth 57–8
and grief 93–4
and Fire 58–9
and Metal 54–7
and Water 59–61

Author Index